Aromatherapy for Practitioners

T0316185

Ulla-Maija Grace's

Aromatherapy
for Practitioners

INDEX COMPILED BY
LYN GREENWOOD

SAFFRON WALDEN
THE C.W. DANIEL COMPANY LIMITED

First published in Great Britain in 1996
by The C.W.Daniel Company Limited
1 Church Path, Saffron Walden
Essex, CB10 1JP, United Kingdom

© Ulla-Maija Grace 1996

ISBN 0 85207 293 7

Reprinted 2000

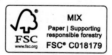

Printed and bound in Great Britain by Clays Ltd, St Ives PLC

Produced in association with
Book Production Consultants plc, Cambridge
Typeset by Cambridge Photosetting Services

Contents

DEDICATION

This book is dedicated to the love that permits and carries all life on this beautiful planet Earth. May the love help us to understand the responsibility that we have for the Earth's wellbeing and all that inhabit it.

My deep, heartfelt thanks to Teuvo for his encouragement and Elina for her patience in deciphering the text.

Introduction

This book has been growing within me for many years. It has been collected from information gained from my very well respected teachers, **Patricia Davis, Pierre Franchomme, Dr. Daniel Penoel** and **Swami Dharmananda Saraswati**, from the many books ploughed through over the years, but most of all from my experiences as a therapist and a teacher. This book therefore is also a heartfelt thanks to all of my teachers – those already mentioned and my clients and students who each have been in their uniqueness the greatest teachers of all.

The importance of writing this book suddenly became very acute when the Persian Gulf War covered the sky with black smoke and pollution, because of man's greed and hatred, putting the fragile environment of the Earth in such danger. The waters were black with oil, suffocating the fish and trapping and killing the birds. It made me feel very deeply sad for the plants, the animals, the Earth as well as the people of this planet. I became aware of the fact that activities of man are and have been a real threat to the purity of the essential oils that we use in aromatherapy. How long will we be able to harvest plants that have at least some right to be called pure and natural? Do we as inhabitants of the Earth understand the importance of the quality of our environment, our food, and the medicines we use for our health and wellbeing?

As an aromatherapist the best way that I may have some influence on bringing this awareness to people is through my work as a therapist, as a teacher and now as an author.

During the years of my involvement in the world of aromatherapy, as a therapist and then as a teacher of aromatherapy, I have become aware of the different levels of training in aromatherapy. At the first meeting of the International Federation of Aromatherapists (IFA) it was decided that a standard of training be set. Over the years, for various reasons, this has been changed many times. New organisations are born from almost every school and no one organisation knows what the students are being taught. Variety is a good thing, and the magnitude of aromatherapy can embrace all the individual philosophies.

This book is designed for all aromatherapists, for those seeking treatment from a qualified aromatherapist, and everyone interested in aromatherapy in general.

Within this book is laid out the basic framework, which I teach and feel to be the very minimum of understanding that the therapist should have of the essential oils and their uses, the carrier oils, client-therapist communication, and themselves as therapists. I also feel that no aromatherapist or any kind of therapist should work without the proper knowledge of anatomy and physiology, as well as an understanding of the more common diseases. All aromatherapists know that aromatherapy is the BEST therapy, but so do all other therapists of their own therapies.

This is fine as long as we know that no one form of therapy is the best for everyone, and that with thorough training and professionalism all therapies and treatments have their place in helping mankind to grow in physical strength and spiritual integrity.

As you read this book you will see that aromatherapy encompasses and embraces all the current forms of treatment given to people. This will help you understand why I see aromatherapy as: 1) a bond between orthodox medicine and homoeopathy in its chemistry and energetics,

2) a connector for psychiatric medicine and therapies assisting in the process of self awareness and understanding, and 3) a physiological link in the touch therapies where each form of manipulation can benefit from the use of essential oils.

Ulla-Maija Grace

1 History and Background to Aromatherapy

The history of the essential oils can be said to be the history of medicine. Throughout the history of humanity aromatic plants have been used to treat man at all levels of his being and existence. Many books cover the history of aromatherapy from different angles; here the approach is from yet another direction.

Yarrow has been found from the burial mounds of prehistoric times and its descendants *Achillea millefolium* and *Achillea liqustica* can be used for aromatherapy as well as herbal medicine. Then it was probably used as a strengthening herb as well as being smoked. In Finnish herbal lore it has names such as 'old women's tobacco' possibly as it is said to help with women's lower back pain. Used internally as a herb it is helpful for varicose veins and haemorrhoids.

The Australian aborigines have used the numerous species of both the *Eucalyptus* and *Melaleuca* in their medicine. The *Melaleuca* oils, such as Tea-tree, have only fairly recently found their way into modern aromatherapy, but have been very extensively studied and researched since their discovery.

Written records of aromatic substances can be found from 4000–2000 years BC. The oldest distillation apparatus, which was found in Pakistan, is approximately 5000 years old. Early historical records describe and classify uses of aromatic plants for example in the following ways:

Anxiety and phobias – *Salvia sclarea, Salvia officinalis, Citrus aurantium* Bigarade flowers, and *Origanum majorana.*

As aromatherapists of today we can accept these. But *Rosmarinus officinalis*, which also is included in this same list, seems rather a surprise until we remember that in excessive doses the stimulating effect of rosemary reverses and becomes sedating. This is probably due to the action of the ketones on the nervous system.

Depression – *Lavandula angustifolia, Zingiber officinale, Chamaemelum nobile* and *Coriandrum sativum*

Once again we can easily accept the lavender and chamomile in this group but might feel a little uneasy about the ginger and coriander. For these we need to consider the many natures of depression and its causes and remember that both coriander and ginger are used for general asthenia and nervous exhaustion.

Insomnia – *Melissa officinalis, Lavandula angustifolia, Citrus aurantium* Bigarade flowers, *Rosmarinus officinalis* and *Thymus vulgaris*.

Melissa, lavender, neroli and, in the light of the above, rosemary are recognisable for this use in today's aromatherapy, but what about the thyme? I have not found a clear answer to this so can only assume that as it has many anti-infectious properties it could ease insomnia by, for example, clearing a respiratory infection.

Difficulties in concentrating – *Eugenia caryophyllus, Citrus aurantium ssp. Bergamia, Ocimum basilicum, Cananga odorata*.

In this list ylang ylang is a little confusing for this purpose but maybe its ability to bring peace to a restless mind can be considered to help concentration.

Hippocrates (460–377 BC) records uses of saffron, thyme, cumin, peppermint and marjoram. The knowledge of these came from the Indian Ayurvedic medicine via the Arabian spice traffic. He also used styrax, myrrh and frankincense *per fumum* as smoke or steam. The literature left by him and his students includes the most important principle of modern natural medicine: 'Above all the purpose of a doctor is to awaken the natural healing energies within the body.'

Ali Hussein Ibn Abdulla Ibn Sina (980–1037 AD) known as **Avicenna** is said to be a very important person in the history of aromatherapy, and his credits are listed in most books of aromatherapy. He was a genius as a child and knew the Koran by heart at the age of 10. He was born in Buhara which now is part of Uzbekistan. In one of my foundation classes many years ago in Finland, there sat, right in the front, a gentleman who clearly was not of Finnish origin. During the lesson we came to a point where I introduced Avicenna as I always did as a very important Arab...immediately the gentleman started frantically waving his hand at me saying "Madam, please Madam, Avicenna was not an Arab. He was Persian, a very wise and civilised person..." Being Persian himself this gentleman had studied herbal lore in his own country and wanted this mistake rectified. Since then I have introduced Avicenna as a Persian.

In addition to the plants already mentioned we can recognise chamomile, juniper and cinnamon from the plants Avicenna used. Of these *Matricaria recutita* is still accepted as part of the medical pharmacopoeia in many countries.

The Arabians began to describe chemical reactions and create nomenclature for chemical substances such as alcohol, alkaloid, aldehyde, syrup, and methods of handling and preparation terms such as distillation, crystallisation via evaporation, filtering etc.

The term *Quintessence* sometimes used when talking about essential oils comes from **Theopharastus Bombastus Von Hohenheim** (1494–1541) known as **Paracelsus**. He discarded all the old theories of medicine and stressed the importance of natural living as a means of preventing and healing illness. He spoke of the 'inner doctor' – a life force, which we need to support our well-being. He brought chemistry into medicine and studied medicinal plants believing that God has made a healing plant for every illness. His search was for the one healing component in each medicinal plant which he called the quintessence.

Carolus Linneaus (1707–1778, **Carl von Linné**) was a professor of medicine in the University of Uppsala, Sweden, and an expert in medicinal plants. He was particularly knowledgeable about the effects of lifestyle on health. Linné's definition of health was:

> "SANITAS: Integra, cui nulla functio corporis persentitu. Corpus agile. Respiratio libera. Facies nitida. Calor universalis. Pulsus magnus aequalis. Somnus placidus. Mens tranquilla."

> "HEALTH: A wholeness, in which no functions of the body are felt. Flexible body. Free respiration. Glowing face. Overall warmness. Great, regular heartbeat. Restful sleep. Tranquil mind."

What more could a person want? Perhaps a spirit that is true and loving towards all humanity and life.

In the history of aromatherapy this century it is said that the father of modern aromatherapy is René Gattefossé, a French chemist, whose family worked in a perfumery. It was Gattefosse who first used the term aromatherapy and published his first thesis of "Aromatherapy" in 1928. He also wrote several scientific papers and other books relating to the use of the essential oils.

During and after the second world war a French medical doctor, **Jean Valnet** used essences in the treatment of many conditions. He wrote a book on aromatherapy in 1964, *The Practice of Aromatherapy*, on his findings in the uses of the essential oils. This book is stilled considered important in the aromatherapy world.

Around the same time as Doctor Valnet, a biochemist **Madame Marguerite Maury** was researching the use of the essential oils for therapeutic and cosmetic purposes. She used massage as the basis for his medical/cosmetic therapy, and made a study of the way in which the aromatic essences work in the physical body, the mind and also on the skin. Her well known book *Secrets of Life and Youth* was published in 1964. Her natural skin care knowledge appears to be largely based on ancient Indian and Chinese information. The current trend of aromatherapy in England has its origins as much in Madam Maury's work as Doctor Valnet's studies into the use of essential oils.

Today there is a great bank of information on the use and properties of the essential oils due to recent studies conducted by several people. The scientific works of **Pierre Franchomme** and **Dr. Daniel Penoel** are of great importance. Their knowledge, experience and intuitive insight into the essential oils and their physical and subtle uses, profoundly aid the path to combining modern science with the intuition of the old sciences.

Their book *L'Aromatherapie, exactement* is currently the most informative and complete work available on aromatherapy.

2 The Approach to Aromatherapy

There are three clearly definable branches of aromatherapy, based on the training of the therapist and the way in which the essential oils are used.

These are cosmetic, medical and therapeutic. In *cosmetic aromatherapy* the therapist is trained as a beautician, with an additional short training section on the uses of aromatic substances for cosmetic massage and caring for the skin. Very often these cosmetic aromatherapy treatments are given using ready blended, prepared oils, possibly defined for relaxation, stimulation or for the various skin types. This type of aromatherapy does not necessarily use natural essential oils, but may also use synthetically prepared aromatic substances. This is a cosmetic beauty treatment for caring for the skin on the face and on the body.

The second form of aromatherapy, "*Aromatic Medicine*", is used by General Practitioners. Naturally this kind of medical aromatherapy demands medical training. On the whole the essential oils are used internally. Essential oils are prescribed to the patient and prepared for internal use by the pharmacist who is trained in this kind of work. This form of treatment is not widely available at the moment because there are very few doctor aromatherapists or pharmacists trained in preparing essential oils for internal use. Like Allopathic Medicine, Aromatic Medicine is directed at specific symptoms and illnesses, where medical knowledge is a necessity.

The third type of aromatherapy is the *Therapeutic Aromatherapy*, which is the focus of this book. From here on, the words therapeutic aromatherapy will be used to cover such titles given to aromatherapy as clinical, classical, and holistic. In therapeutic aromatherapy the essential oils are applied to the body in various ways, most important of which is massage. Other methods are inhalations, perfumes, compresses, sprays, baths, etc. The olfactory system is of great important in therapeutic aromatherapy treatments.

The problems treated by therapeutic aromatherapy vary from the everyday, basic aches and pains to more complex and chronic conditions, e.g. arthritis. Most stress-related problems are very successfully treated with aromatherapy. Some of the essential oils have powerful antibacterial and antiviral properties and can be used to treat such infections as occur from viral, bacterial or fungal infestations of the body. Some essential oils contain plant hormones or influence the endocrine system in such a way that these can be used to help with problems related to the menstrual cycle. The aromatherapist of today can draw on the knowledge of distant historical wisdom as well as modern scientific findings.

Every aromatherapist should embrace the old and the new approaches, the scientific, the empirical and the intuitive. Each one has its values. Each one has its uses. To know only the science, or to feel that by knowing the science one's ability to work in the old way and to develop one's intuition will be depleted, causes something of the true nature of aromatherapy to be lost. One has to go hand in hand with the other, especially as the need for higher qualifications and training in all fields of alternative and complementary medicine is becoming increasingly important. It is a great responsibility and privilege to be allowed and able to help somebody and to assist them in improving their health. Without the knowledge of either anatomy and physiology, or the thorough understanding of the essential oils, the respect that needs to be given to each client, as an inherent part of the art of aromatherapy, will be lost.

Dr. Dietrich Gumbel has studied the ecology of the earth, plants and man and divides the effect of the essential oils into three areas of man's existence:

> The effect of the essential oils on the nervous system is in the energetic function of the body and is therefore at the level of the spirit of man.

> The effect of the essential oils on the emotional level works on the blood and fluid circulation of the body and the soul/feelings level of man.

> The hormonal effects of the essential oils work as biocatalysts on the intercellular function on the physical body.

Thus, according to Dr. Gumbel, the essential oils work on all levels of human existence; the physical, the emotional or soul and the spirit. Aromatherapy as a holistic form of treatment is best illustrated using a triangle.

Grouping the various forms of treatment in the corners of the triangle according to their field of approach leaves aromatherapy in the centre of the triangle. It has the *manipulating* features and the benefits it brings in the form

AROMATHERAPY IN RELATION TO OTHER THERAPIES

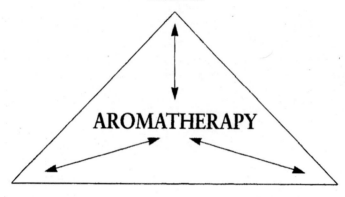

Psychiatry
Psychology
Psychosynthesis
Homoeopathy
Counselling therapies
all treatments that aim to
influence the mind and psyche

**PSYCHOLOGICAL
THERAPIES**

AROMATHERAPY

**MANIPULATIVE
THERAPIES**
Physiotherapy
Osteopathy
Chiropractic treatment
Massage therapies
All treatments that
manipulate the muscular
structure

**INTERNAL
THERAPIES**
Allopathic medicine
Eastern medicine
Herbalism
Homoeopathy
Nutritional therapies
Vitamin and mineral treatments
Fasting
All orally prescribed medicines

of massage. It has *internal* uses, as the essential oils have a fine molecular structure which allows them to be absorbed into the bloodstream through the skin and via the respiratory tract, into the lungs, from where they are absorbed into the blood stream. The *psychological* effect of the essential oils is initially through the olfactory system. The sense of smell has an immediate effect upon the emotions and mood of the person being treated which also causes physiological changes. The use of massage has a deeply relaxing, calming effect on the mind, through touch. Stimulating the nerve endings of the whole of the skin leads to a deeply relaxed physical and mental state. The psychological effect is enhanced by the nurturing and caring attitude of the therapist, which is of the utmost importance in aromatherapy. Aromatherapy embraces man as a whole and the treatments are aimed at the whole person. **Dr. Edward Bach,** who developed the Bach Flower Remedies, said 'treat the person not the disease.'

In aromatherapy treatment also means using the material, the essential oils as a whole. The best essential oils for therapy, no doubt, come from growing conditions that are as close to natural as possible. Wholeness also means that the distillation time for the oil is long enough to extract as much of the therapeutic properties of the oils from the plant material as is possible.

3 Essential Oils

THE IMPORTANCE OF QUALITY

The Plant

Naturally, the plant itself is an essential and vital part of aromatherapy; the quality of the plant is extremely important.

Is man in his greed and arrogance destroying the Earth? Is he separating and withdrawing himself from the rest of nature? Methods of growing and cultivation are forced and unnatural, creating an unhealthy environment for plants, where they are vulnerable to pests and diseases. Pests and diseases are destroyed by the use of chemicals. The methods of cultivation not only create unhealthy plants, which we feed to our animals and ourselves, but also destroy the natural ecology of the Earth for future generations. Eventually the chemicals used can be found in our bodies. It is not surprising that the animals, the plants, the Earth and ourselves all suffer from unbeatable and new diseases.

When choosing and using essential oils it is vital that we use oils that have been acquired from plants that are either grown wild, in their natural environment, or that they have been cultivated in a natural way without chemical pesticides and fertilisers in areas that are as free from air pollutants as possible. Our bodies are already under great strain trying to cope with the general pollutants in our environment. Therefore when we are unwell, we should not burden our body systems further with chemically polluted essential oils (through cultivation or adulteration).

Several studies have shown that the effects of the soil and growing conditions of the plants have a profound effect on the quality of the essential oil they produce. The effect and quality of light is also very important in the production of the various aromatic molecules in the plant.

9

Checking the quality of the plants used for Herbal Remedies and the Essential Oils for Pharmacological and Therapeutic purposes

1. Quality
   - Organoleptic examination of the plant
   - Appearance, taste, smell
2. Identification
   - Macroscopic – ground plant
   - Microscopic – oil containers typical for the plant
   - Chemical reactions – TLC (thin layer chromatography)
   - Other chemical reactions – chromatography
3. Purity
   - Loss of dry weight
   - Examination of ashes
   - Substances not soluble in acids
4. Chemical Composition
   - Mass spectography, gas chromatography
5. Microbiological Findings
   - Bacteria
   - Fungi
   - Moulds
   - Pathogenic microbes
6. Pesticides and Others
   - During growth
   - During storage
   - Radioactive substances

This is the standard checking procedure for plants and oils used for medical, therapeutic and food preparation.

PARTS OF THE PLANT USED

The essential oils can occur in practically every part of a plant. For example, in the flowers of jasmine, rose and orange, the leaves of sage, eucalyptus, lavender and rosemary, the seeds of parsley and dill, the rind of the citrus fruits, the bark of cinnamon, the resin of myrrh and frankincense, the stems of wood such as rosewood and sandalwood, the root of angelica and ginger, in the berries of juniper and the whole plant above ground of geranium.

The plant material contains very small amounts of essence. Rose only contains 0.02% of the weight of the plant material compared to lavender and rosemary at a much higher percentage of 2% and some even higher than 2%. It is this very concentration that makes essential oils different from other herbal and plant remedies. Essential oils should not be used undiluted. They work very well in combinations with other forms of plant remedies, such as herb teas, tinctures and macerations.

Essential oils are made by the plant in specialised glands. The epidermic gland is situated on the outer surface of the leaves. Plant families such as Verbenaceae, Lamiaceae and Rosaceae have this type of essence-producing glands. These plants are easily recognizable by simply brushing the leaves of the plant; because the gland is exposed on the surface of the leaf it readily emits the essence and aroma which is immediately noticeable.

The schizogene gland occurs, for example, in plant families such as Myrtaceae, Hypericaceae and Rutaceae. In plants such as Eucalyptus and *Hypericum perforatum*, the gland is situated within the leaf itself and is no longer exposed to the air. The schizogene gland also occurs in woody substances in a different formation, e.g. the Santalaceae, Abietaceae and Lauraceae families. With these one needs first to break the wood of the plant finely before the oil can be extracted from it.

The molecules produced by the gland as well as the liquid in the storing sack is called *essence*. These specific glands in the plant only manufacture the aromatic molecules, never any other compounds.

EXTRACTION OF THE ESSENTIAL OIL

The most commonly used method of processing the plant material into essential oil is steam distillation. In this method water vapour (steam) is passed through the plant material at varying pressures and temperatures, and in passing through the steam extracts the volatile aromatic molecules and carries them through a cooling pipe into a container where the separation of the cooled steam (water) and the essential oils takes place. So, within the plant there is the *essence* and after distillation, after processing, the *essential oil*. The composition of this essence is not exactly the same as the essential oil, as changes, chemical reactions occur during the processing of the plant material. The heat, the water and the oxygen have an influence on the essence and change its structure. Some of the more volatile particles will disappear and sometimes new compounds are made during the process of distillation, e.g. matricine in *Matricaria recutita* changes into chamazulene.

The distillation time for therapeutic oils is much longer than the distillation in the perfume industry. This will be reflected in the aroma and the price. The perfume oils are not useful for therapeutic purposes as they do not contain all the possible components. An older method of distillation which is now rarely used is direct distillation, where the plant material is heated in water and the steam is collected and cooled in the same way as in steam distillation. For more delicate plants and flowers vacuum distillation is used where steam at a lower temperature is passed through the plant material. This gentler method helps to preserve the delicate aroma of the flower.

A very old and laborious method of extraction is enfleurage, in which the petals are spread on a layer of fat. As the essence gets absorbed into the fat the petals are removed and replaced by a new layer of petals. This process is repeated until the fat can absorb no more of the essence. The mixture of essence and the fat is then agitated in alcohol.

Some oils are extracted by a direct cold processing, such as the rinds of citrus fruits like lemon and orange. In effect these are still in the state of the essence as no heat or water is used for their extraction. The fruits used for aromatherapy purposes on the skin should, without exception, be produced **without pesticides or other protecting agents**. The reason for this of course is that any and all such substances will be left in the essence and be a potential cause for allergic reaction or other irritation.

The latest form of extraction is carbon dioxide extraction. This method has only been in use for a very short time and is not commonly used at the moment due to the high cost of the equipment.

UNDERSTANDING THE STRUCTURE OF THE OILS

The substance that is extracted from the plant as essential oil is called essence whilst still within the plant. It has some very specific functions for the plant. The word itself means that it is necessary for life:

* In the pathology of the plant, the essence fights infections and moulds.
* Protects the plant after damage from drying or infection, e.g. resin, which is a phenolic compound.

Essential 'oils' are not actually oils, but they behave like oils in some ways. They do not dissolve in water, but float on top of it. They blend well with vegetable oils and alcohol. The aromatic molecules in the essential oils have varying degrees of volatility.

Essential oils are complex blends of carbon (C), hydrogen (H) and oxygen (O). Hydrogen occurs in the sun, the stars and on the Earth, and is part of water. Oxygen is breathed in by animals and man and given out by plants, a mutual need, a mutual cycle. Carbon is the basis of organic compounds. Light equals life. In the plant, chlorophyll harvests the energy of the sun and uses this in the process of photosynthesis to make foods/sugars, which all humans and animals depend on. This process is also the beginning of the formation of the aromatic molecules.

The majority of the aromatic molecules are based on the terpenic structure composed of isoprene chains of 5 carbons. There are very few aromatic molecules of more than 20 carbons. The essential oils are formed through two routes of plant metabolism. Most common of these is the terpenic group. The second group contains the phenols, coumarins etc. The aromatic molecules that have no oxygen content are called terpenes. Through the process of oxidation (adding OH) and reduction (removing H) alcohols, aldehydes, ketones, esters, lactones, and acids are formed.

There are some essential oils in which a great proportion of the components are of one type, such as, *Betula alleghaniensis* (98% methyl salicylate) or *Aniba rosaeodora* (95% linalol). At the other end of the scale there are essential oils with a multitude of different molecules, for example, *Pelargonium × asperum* and the various roses. These have in excess of 250 known compounds and a number of 'unknowns'. Within each species of plant there can be several chemotypes e.g. in Finland 22 different CT's of *Tanacetum vulgare* can be found growing wild. It is therefore important to know the composition of the essential oils used for therapeutic purposes. This can be revealed by paper chromatography or by gas-chromatography.

For a new essential oil, a method known as mass spectrography is used first to determine its molecular composition. The various constituents are recorded and form a basic 'map' against which to check future distillations.

Pierre Franchomme discovered and mapped the electro-polarity of the various aromatic molecules. This was made possible by the creation of a device in which the essential oil is broken down into a very fine aerosol mist of individual molecules. The energy or charge, created by each molecule, is transmitted to a recording device, which indicates whether it is a positive or negative electrical charge. The negative molecules have an excess of electrons and are therefore electron donors, whereas the positive molecules have an electron deficiency and readily accept electrons.

Although the essential oils do not dissolve in water, there are some particles of the oils that are more readily water soluble than others. The further the oxidation process goes the more water soluble the particle becomes and the less fat soluble. This means that terpenes are the most fat and least water soluble components in the essential oil. This solubility structure has a bearing on the route and speed of absorption, through skin and respiration.

Using these two types of polarity, the electro positivity/negativity and the water solubility poles of the essential oils, Pierre Franchomme created a reference chart in which he gives an overall polarity classification for the essential oils. As a rule, those essential oils that are mainly in the negative pole of the chart have a relaxing, calming effect and those at the positive pole are more stimulating and tonic in their action. This knowledge of the polarity of the molecules can be used actively in aromatherapy.

These classifications can, to a certain extent, also be looked at in the light of the Chinese tradition, the negative and cooling aspect as Yin and the positive, warming aspect as Yang; the apolar as being dry and the polar as wet. The main groups of the aromatic molecules are: Terpenes, Phenols, Alcohols, Oxides, Acids, Aromatic aldehydes, Coumarins, Lactones, Ketones, Aldehydes, Esters and Phenyl-methyl-ethers. Each group has a general property for which it can be applied in the treatments, and within each group there are specific molecules with very special properties. (See chart on page 15)

List of Abbreviations used in this Book

- ENE = terpene
- OL = alcohol
- ONE = ketone
- YLE = ester
- AL = aldehyde
- OX = oxide
- PME = phenyl-methyl-ether
- COUM = coumarin
- LACT = lactone
- AROM AL = aromatic aldehyde

C10 and C15 = mono- and sesquiterpenes
C10, C15 and C20 = mono-, sesqui- and diterpenols

By putting the components and their percentages in the appropriate circles, the chart on page 18 can be used to define the balance of each oil when the composition of the essential oil is known. This will give a basic reference for the uses of the oil according to its structure and also in terms of the temperaments as described later in the book (page 137).

General Properties of the Aromatic Molecule Groups

Each of the molecular groups has a general function, and some molecules of
a group can have specific function or purpose as a therapeutic substance.

Molecule	General Function and Property	Examples of Specific Function
Terpene C + H	• non water-soluble	

Monoterpene
C10 contains
    10 carbon atoms
	• air antiseptic
	• general antiseptic
		Picea mariana
		Pinus sylvestris
		cortisone-like
		Pinenes
		• lymphotonic and
		decongestant
		Terebinthene
		• very powerful general
		    stimulant
		Juniperus species
		• stimulate renal
		    activity

Sesquiterpene
C15 contains
    15 carbon atoms
	• non water-soluble
	• general antiseptic
		Chamazulene
		• anti-allergic
		• antispasmodic
		• anti-inflammatory
		• cicatrisant
		• influences ovarian
		    function via the
		    pituitary
		Zingiberene
		• choleretic
		• antihepatotoxic
		• relieves nausea

Alcohol = terphene + OH monoterpenols C10	• general and nerve tonic • anti-infectious • bactericide • fungicide • parasiticide	

Sesquiterpenols C15 and Diterpenols C20 Phenols	• venous and lymphatic decongestant • some anti-infectious action	Viridiflorol • oestrogen-like • phlebotonic Cedrol • phlebotonic Santalol • cardiotonic • antispetic action in the urinary tract
	• tonic and stimulant • anti-infectious, stronger than monoterpenols • bactericide • viricide • fungicide • parasiticide • dermocaustic	Thymol, carvacrol • immunostimulant
Aldehyde = 1* Alcohol – H terpenci aldehyde	• litholytic • local anti inflammatory • calming of the nervous system	
Aromatic aldehyde	• mucous membrane irritant	
Ketone = 2* alcohol – H	• cicatrisant • potentially neurotoxic • mucolytic esp. of the respiratory tract and the female genitalia • lipolytic	
Lactone	• mucolytic • expectorant • can cause allergic reactions on skin	
Acid = aldehyde + OH		Salicylic acid • anti-inflammatory Citronellic acid • stimulant of hepatocellular activity

Ester = acid + –OL	• antispasmodic • calming • anti-inflammatory	The area of the antispasmodic and calming actions are directly related to the structure of the ester. Terpenyle acetate • intestinal Benzyle acetate
Coumarins	• sedative and calming of central nervous system • hypnotic • anticonvulsive when combined with esters and ethers • furocoumarins and pyrocoumarins are photosensitizing	These are visnadine, psoralene, bergaptol bergaptene phellopterine angelisine pimpinelline
Phenols Methyl-ethers	• antispasmodic • in large doses stupefying	Anethole • oestrogen-like Estragole = Chavicol ME • antispasmodic Eugenol MR • local anaesthetic
Ether-oxides	• tonic and stimulant • antispasmodic	Myristicine • stupefying • hallucinogenic • abortifacient
Phthalides	• stimulate the detoxification of liver	
Oxides	• stimulate the secretions of the exocrine glands • expectorant	Dioxides • antiparisitic

ELECTRO-POLARITY AND GENERAL PROPERTIES
OF THE ESSENTIAL OILS

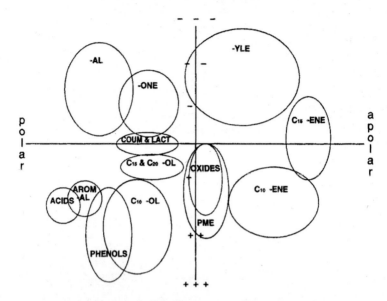

Reproduced with the kind permission of Pierre Franchomme

Special Points for the Aromatherapist to note on the use of Essential Oils

I *MEDICATION*

Where there are references in the applications section for definite medical conditions they are there for information. These should act as a guide as to when **not to use that particular oil if there is medication in use for that condition.** It is important to be aware of this so as **not to throw the medication into imbalance** e.g. HRT, thyroid, diabetes etc.

II *BABIES*

My opinion is that essential oils should not be used on babies as a matter of routine, for example for nappy rash. Carrier oils, like almond, are quite often sufficient. For irritability and sleep disorders, baths in herbal teas, or a drop or two in a burner in the room are effective. If there is need to use essential oils directly on the baby's skin, for example for infection, gentle oils such as *Aniba rosaeodora* or *Thymus vulgaris ct linalol* in 1/6th of the adult dose should suffice. Babies and young children respond to the chemical, the energetic and the informative aspects of the essential oils very strongly, hence doses and use should reflect this.

III PREGNANCY

Contrary to most current information on the use of essential oils during pregnancy, I hold a very strong opinion **against this use**. Pregnancy is not an illness and as such does not need treatment as a matter of course. We have enough scientific knowledge on the effects of the essential oils to avoid unnecessary use during pregnancy. There are naturally no studies of these effects on the unborn, as no mother with sufficient awareness would take part in such a study. Therefore, we can only base our judgement on the known effects of the oils.

We know the oils are absorbed through the skin into the bloodstream and through the placenta into the baby. **We know** the essential oils influence cellular metabolism, increase the regeneration of cutaneous cells, influence the immune system, have hormonal activities, to name but a few. Do we want to take the responsibility of the effect of these oils on the developing new human being? Do we know how this will effect the future life of that child?

LACTATION

The use of the essential oils during lactation should also be avoided for the above reasons. Oils will affect the baby through the mother's milk.

IV CHILDREN AND THE ELDERLY

The doses for children and the elderly need to be reduced to about half or one third of the adult dose depending on the size of the child and the condition of the elderly person. Through experience I have found that as older people often have had illnesses of many kinds and have had to use strong medication, their bodies cannot tolerate strong doses. Excessive use of essential oils can cause powerful reactions and cleansing processes on both the physical and emotional levels. The choice of oils for the elderly has to be carefully considered. Some of the gentle oils such as *Aniba rosaeodora*, are always well received as is also citrus aurantium flowers.

Children on the other hand need only low doses due to the purity and size of their bodies and their sensitivity to the actions of the oils. The use of essential oils that contain ketones or have hormonal activity should be avoided.

DOSAGE

Massage:		
Adults	2–3% = 2–3 drops/5ml	
Elderly/Children	1–1.5%	
Children 2–7 yrs.	no more than 0.5%	
Babies	—	
Steam inhalation	2–4 drops	
Baths	6–8 drops	
Foot/hand	2–4 drops	
Hot and cold compresses	4 drops	On a cotton or linen cloth. Avoid direct contact of diluted oil on skin
Pot pourri/burner	4+ drops	
Skin care products	0.5–1%	
Perfumes	25–100%	Not daily use on skin.

Please note:
The individual properties of the oils effect the dosage.

Drops used are calculated on dropper size that averages 160–190 drops per 5ml, with the exception of very viscous oils, e.g. *Santalum album*.

ESSENTIAL OILS IN ALPHABETICAL ORDER

In the following pages you will find 42 essential oils. In my experience applications marked with an * are their most important uses

LATIN NAME	ENGLISH NAME
Achillea liqustica	Yarrow
Angelica Archangelica	Angelica
Aniba rosaeodora	Rosewood
Artemesia dracunculus	Tarragon
Artemisia arborescence	Great Mugwort
Betula alleghaniensis	Yellow Birch
Boswellia carterit	Frankincense/Olibanum
Cananga odorata forma genuina	Ylang ylang / Flower of flowers
Cedrus atlantica	Cedarwood
Chamaemelum nobile	Roman chamomile
Citrus aurantium – ssp. bergamia	Bergamot
Citrus limon	Lemon
Citrus reticulata	Mandarin
Citrus aurantium ssp. aurantium	Neroli bigarade/orange flower/orange leaf Petitgrain

Commiphora molmol	Myrrh
Cupressus sempervirens	Cypress
Cymbopogon martinii – var motia	Indian Palmarosa
Eucalyptus globulus	Eucalyptus globulus
Eucalpytus citriodora	Citrus scented Eucalyptus
Eucalyptus radiata	Xeucalyptus Australiana
Foeniculum vulgare var dulce	Fennel
Helychrysum italicum ssp. serotinum	Italian Everlasting
Junpiterus communis ssp. communis	Juniper
Juniperus communis var. montana	Juniper
Lavandula spica / lavandula latifolia	Spiked Lavender
Lavandula angustifolia	True Lavender
Matricaria recutita	German or blue chamomile
Melaleuca quinquenervia – viridiflorol	Niaouli
Melaleuca alternifolia	Tea-tree
Mentha × piperita	Peppermint
Ocimum basilicum – var. basilicum	Basil
Origanum majorana	Sweet Marjoram
Pelargonium × asperum	Geranium
Picea mariana	Black Spruce
Pinus sylvestris	Scotch Pine
Ravensara aromatica	Ravensara
Rosmarinum pyramidalis	Rosemary
Salvia sclarea	Clary Sage
Santalum album	Sandalwood
Thymus vulgaris ct. linaloliferum	Common Thyme
Zingiber officinale	Ginger

ESSENTIAL OILS FOR EMOTIONAL CONDITIONS

Angelica archangelica	Angelica
Aniba rosaeodora	Rosewood
Boswellia carterii	Frankincense/Olibanum
Canaga odorata	Ylang ylang
Chamaemelum nobile	Roman Chamomile
Citrus aurantium ssp. bergamia	Bergamot
Citrus aurantium ssp. aurantium neroli	Orange flower
Citrus paradisi	Grapefruit
Citrus reticulata	Mandarin
Jasminum officinale	Jasmine
Melissa officinalis	Melissa Balm
Rosa damascena	Rose
Santalum album	Sandalwood
Vetiveria zizanoides	Vetiver

ANGELICA

Angelica archangelica

Apiaceae
(Umbelliferae)

Part used – roots

Note – Base

Main components
Monoterpenes (about 73%): Phellandrene, alpha– (24%) and beta-pinenes, limonene
Esters: bornyle acetate
Coumarins: umbelliferone, archangelicine, angelicine, bergaptene

Properties
Anticoagulant
Anti-inflammatory
Carminative
Cardio tonic
Hormone-like
Sedative

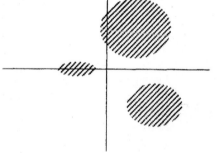

Applications
Anorexia
Any problems related to
stress, such as anxiety, nervous fatigue, flatulence
Insomnia
Spasmodic enterocolitis
Thickening of blood

Contra-indications
Photosensitizing due to the furocoumarins and bergaptene
Angelica archangelia – all parts of the plant are fragrant. The essential oils on the market are either from the seeds or the roots. Angelica has a reputation for being especially good for female disorders.

Experiential note
This is a very calming and soothing oil. Aids sleep when used in massage even in very small doses.

BASIL

Ocimum basilicum – var. basilicum

Labiatae
(Labiatae)
Note – Top

Parts used – leaves and flowering tops

Main components
Monoterpenols: linalol, fenchol, alpha-terpineol, citronellol
Esters: fenchyle acetate, linalyl acetate
Phenols: eugenol
Phenols ME: chavicol methyl-ether (85–88%)
Oxides: cineole
Ketones: about 1%

Properties
Antibacterial
Anti-depressant
Anti-infectious
Anti-inflammatory
*Antispasmodic
Cephalic
Regulator and tonic of
the nervous system

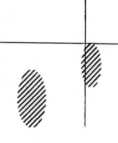

Applications
Anxiety
Circulatory problems in veins
*Constipation
Decongestant of veins
Depression
*Dysmenorrhoea
*Exhaustion
Gastritis
Insect repellent
Prostatitis
Rheumatoid polyarthritis
Spasmodic gastroenteritis
Urinary infections
Varicose veins

23

Contra-indications
No known contra-indications, though can cause irritation of skin if sensitive.

Experiential note
* The antispasmodic activity of this oil is especially good for muscular spasms, and spasms in the intestine and the bowel.
* Stimulates and clears thinking processes – excellent for keeping alert.
* A blend for long-distance drivers to use as an inhalant (e.g. on a handkerchief) Bergamot/Basil/Thyme Thujanol.

BERGAMOT

Citrus aurantium – ssp. bergamia   Rutaceae
Parts used – cold pressed oil from skin of fruit   Note – Top

Main components
The volatile particles:
Monoterpenes: alpha pinene, camphene, limonene
Monoterpenols: Linalol, nerol, geraniol, alpha-terpineol
Esters: linalyl acetate
Aldehydes: citrals
Coumarins: Bergamotine,
bergaptene and others
There are also some non-
volatile particles in this oil

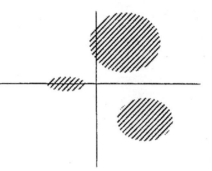

Properties
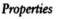
Analgesic
Antibactierial
Antidepressant
Anti-infectious
Antiseptic
Antispasmodic
*Calming and sedating
Tonic in small doses
It is said to be an appetite balancer, deodorant and febrifuge

Applications
Acne
*Agitation
Eczema
Fever
Haemorrhoids
Herpes Simplex
*Infection of the urinary tract
Infections of the mouth
Insomnia
Loss of appetite
Skin care
Spasmodic colitis

The most important areas for this oil are its uses as inhalations for *depression* and *anxiety states*. This is a *balancer of fluctuating moods* and can be refreshing or calming as required. It is a wonderful anti-stress oil, useful to relieve *insomnia, night terrors* and bad dreams.

Contra-indications
This oil is not suitable to be used just before going into sunshine; preferably 72 hours must lapse before sunbathing or using a sunlamp. Makes the skin photosensitive, can cause blotchy tanning.

Experiential note
Calming, uplifting effects appear to become reversed if used simultaneously with alcohol.

IFA compulsory (Meaning that these are the 20 oils that the IFA requires to be read/known for their exam with another 20 oils).

BIRCH – YELLOW

Betula alleghaniensis   Betulaceae
Parts used – bark   Note – Top

Main components
Esters: methyl salicylate 99%

Properties
Analgesic – cutaneous application
Anti-inflammatory
Antispasmodic
Hepato-stimulant

Applications
Arthritis
Cramps
Hypertension
Muscular Rheumatism
Neuralgia (Hiltunen)
Sciatica
Some headaches
Tendonitis
Vaso-dilator

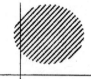

Contra-indications
Caution – lowers blood pressure.

Experiential note
This oil has a very powerful smell and in large doses may be unpleasant. For arthritis blend *Betula alleghaniensis* with *Eucalyptus citriodora* and for headaches, to increase liver function, *Betula alleghaniensis* and *Mentha piperita*.

27

CEDARWOOD

Cedrus atlantica

Abietaceae
(Pinaceae)
Note – Middle

Parts used – wood

Main components
Sesquiterpenes (50%)
Sesquiterpenols (30%): Atlantol
Sesquiterpenones (20%): Alpha- and beta-atlantones

Properties
Cicatrisant
Lipolytic
Lymphotonic

Applications
Bronchitis
Cellulite
Fluid retention

Contra-indications
Babies
Pregnant women
(neurotoxic, abortive)

Experiential note
I find that *Cupressus sempervirens* covers all of the applications of this oil on the physical level. I tend to avoid cedarwood due to its ketone content.

IFA compulsory.

CHAMOMILE – GERMAN OR BLUE

Matricaria recutita

Asteraceae
(Compositae)

Parts used – flowering tops

Note – Middle

Sometimes *Artemisia arborescence* is called Blue Chamomile. It should not be used as a replacement for *Matricaria recutita* as it has a very high ketone content.

Main components
Sesquiterpenes: chamazulene, dihydrochamazulene I & II
Sesquiterpenols: alpha-bisabol
Coumarins: umbelliferone
Oxides: bisabolol oxide

Properties
*Anti-allergic
*Anti-inflammatory
*Antispasmodic
Cicatrisant
Digestive tonic, and eases
digestive problems in general

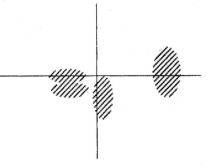

Applications
Amenorrhoea
Cystitis
*Dysmenorrhoea
Dyspepsia
Earache (child) – 1 drop in a carrier on cotton wool
*Eczema
Gastroduodenal ulcers
PMT
*Skin infections
Skin ulcers

Contra-indications
No known contra-indications.

Experiential note
Eases irritation of skin caused by candida albicans.

CHAMOMILE – ROMAN

Chamaemelum nobile/Anthemis nobilis

Asteraceae
(Compositae)

Parts used – flowers

Note – Middle

Main components
Alcohols: transpinocarveol, farnesol
Esters (75-80%): isobutyl angulate (36-40%)
Ketones: pinocarvone
Lactones

Properties
Anti-inflammatory
Antiparasitic
Antispasmodic
*Calming of the central
nervous system*
Febrifuge
Pre-anaesthetic

Applications
Anorexia
Asthma of nervous origin
Digestive problems e.g. dyspepsia, nausea, vomiting
Intestinal parasites
Neuralgia
Neuritis
Pre-operative for calming
Shock

This plant has traditionally been used to treat problems in babies; earache, teething and colic. It has also been used for *aching* and *inflamed muscles, insomnia and anxiety.* Hair rinses for fair hair to give highlights. Skin care and eczema.

Contra-indications
No known contra-indications.

Experiential note
Caution – do not overuse as the calming effect will be reversed. In large doses also causes stimulation of bowel action (laxative effect).

IFA compulsory.

CLARY SAGE

Salvia sclarea

Labiatae
(Labiatae)

Parts used – flower tops and leaves

Note – Middle

Main components
Monoterpenes: camphene, myrcene, limonene, terpinolene
Sesquiterpenes (5%): beta-caryophyllene
Monoterpenols (15%): linalol, terpinene-4-ol, alpha-terpineol,
Citronellol, nerol, geraniol, borneol
Sesquiterpenols: spathulenol
Diterpenols (5%): sclareol
Esters up to 75%: linalyl
acetate 62-75%
Esther: methyl-hexyl-ether
Aldehydes
Oxides: cineole, linalol oxide
Ketones
Coumarins
Bifunctional monoterpenoids

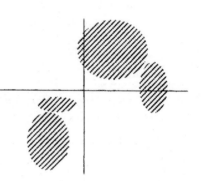

Properties
Antibacterial
Antidiabetic
Anti-epileptic
Anti-infectious
*Antispasmodic
Aphrodisiac
Cholesterol reducing
Cicatrisant
Neurotonic
*Oestrogen-like
*Relaxant
*Sedative

Applications
Amenorrhoea
Circulatory disorders
Depression

Frigidity
Fungal skin infections
Genital infections (due to hormonal imbalances)
Haemorrhoids
Impotence due to stress
Menopausal and premenopausal problems
Muscular spasm and pain
Nervous fatigue
Varicose veins

Contra-indications
Breast mastosis/cystic mastopathy. Not to be used continuously for long periods. Not for young girls' menstrual problems. Cancer. Not for continuous use with HRT. Not for children.

Experiential note
This is an excellent oil for balancing the menstrual cycle. When using oestrogen-like essential oils, follow the natural rhythm, the oestrogen phase, of the menstrual cycle.

IFA compulsory.

CYPRESS

Cupressus sempervirens　　　　　　　　　Cupressaceae
Parts used – needles and twigs　　　　　　Note – Base

Main components
Monoterpenes (70%): alpha-pinene
Sesquiterpenes: alpha-cedrene
Sesquiterpenols: cedrol 7%
Diterpenols labdaniques: manool, sempervirol
Diterpenic acids

Properties
Antibacterial
Anti-infectious
Lymphatic and venous decongestant
Tonic for the nervous and digestive system

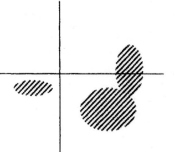

Applications
Cellulite
Coughs (all types)
Enuresis
Exhaustion
Haemorrhoids (internal and external)
Skin care – tonic for oily skin
Varicose veins

Contra-indications
Mastopathy.

Experiential note
A very good oil for varicose veins when used daily, but prolonged use of this oil appears to raise blood pressure in subjects prone to high blood pressure.

IFA compulsory.

EUCALYPTUS – AUSTRALIAN

Eucalyptus Radiata ssp radiata   Myrtaceae
Parts used – leaves   Note – Top

Main components
Monoterpenes: pinenes, mycrene
Monoterpenols: linalol, borneol, terpineols, geraniol
Monoterpenals: myrtenal, citronellal, geranial, neral
Oxides: cineole (62-72%)

Properties
Antibacterial
Anticatarrhal
Anti-inflammatory
Antiseptic particularly for the
respiratory and urinary tracts
Antiviral
Expectorant
Immunostimulant
Stimulating, positive oil

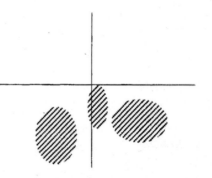

Applications
Acne
Asthenia
Endometriosis
Neuralgia
Otitis
Respiratory infections of all kinds
Sinusitis
Vaginitis

Contra-indications
No known contra-indications. Cineole can cause irritation to some asthma
sufferers.

Eucalyptus radiata has that familiar aroma of eucalyptus sweets. It is
especially good for respiratory disorders, coughs and flu. J. Valnet suggests it
is used for burns and wounds to aid formation of new tissue.

This is a nice oil to use as an antiseptic for the room air in combination with
Eucalyptis globulus or a very good insect repellent.

Experiential note

If an asthma sufferer can tolerate this oil it is very good for clearing the dry, blocked sebaceous glands that appear so often on an asthmatic person's back. It seems to help the skin breathe more freely.

EUCALYPTUS – CITRUS SCENTED

Eucalyptus citriodora   Myrtaceae
Parts used – leaves and twigs   Note – Top

Main components

Monoterpenic alcohols: citronellol 15–20%, trans-pinocarveol, geraniol
Esters: citronellyl acetate, –butyrate and –citronellate
Aldehydes: citronellal 40–80%

Properties

Anti-infectious
Anti-inflammatory
Antispasmodic
*Calming
*Sedative

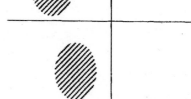

Applications

*Arthritis
Cystitis
Hypertension
*Rheumatism
Vaginitis

Contra-indications

Not for prolonged use if suffering from low blood pressure.

Experiential note

Helps to let go of rigid mental patterns. Very suitable for choleric temperaments. Will reduce dark pigmentation on moles.

IFA compulsory.

EUCALYPTUS – GLOBULUS

Eucalyptus globulus Myrtaceae
Parts used – leaves and twigs Note – Top

Main components
Monoterpenes: pinenes
Sesquiterpenes: aromadendrene
Sesquiterpenols: globulol, ledol
Aldehydes: butyraldehyde, valeraldehyde
Ketones: pinocarvone, carvone
Oxides: cineole 70–75%

Properties
Antiseptic
Antiviral
*Expectorant
General anti-infectious agent
Mucolytic

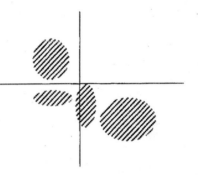

Applications
Adenoiditis
*All respiratory infections
Bacterial and candidal dermatitis
Bronchial asthma

Contra-indications
Babies
Young children

Powerful expectorant due to the high oxide content. Useful for destroying airborne bacteria at times of infections.

IFA compulsory.

FENNEL

Foeniculum vulgare var dulce

Apiaceae
(Umbelliferae)

Parts used – seeds

Note – Top

Main components
Monoterpenes: alpha-pinene, limonene 3.5–18%
Monoterpenols: fenchol
Phenol-menthyl-ethers: chavicol ME 2.8–4%, cis-anethole, trans-anethole 52–70%
Oxides: cineole TR– 6.5%
Ketones: fenchone 0.2–2.6%, camphor 0.3%
Coumarins and furocoumarins; ombelliferone, bergaptene

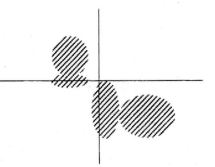

Properties
Antiseptic
Antispasmodic
(neuromuscular)
Carminative
Cardio-tonic
Emmenagogue
Increases appetite
*Oestrogen-like
Tonic and stimulant in small doses
Tonic for the respiratory system
Vermifuge

Applications
Amenorrhoea
Asthma
Dyspepsia
Flatulence
Indigestion
Intestinal parasites
Irregular periods
*Menopausal and premenopausal problems

Palpitations
Spasmodic colitis

Contra-indications
Babies
Pregnant women
Young children
Epilepsy
Photosensitizing – bergaptene

IFA compulsory.

FRANKINCENSE/OLIBANUM

Boswellia carterii
Parts used – oleo gum resin

Burseraceae
Note – Middle

Main components
Monoterpenes: (40%) alpha-pinene, limonene
Sesquiterpenes: alpha-gurjunene
Alcohols: borneol, trans-pinocarveol, farnesol
Bifunctional components: alcohol-ketones; olibanol. Alcohol-oxides; incensoloxide

Properties
Anticatarrhal
Antidepressant
Cicatrisant
Expectorant
Immunostimulant

Applications
Asthma
Bronchitis
Nervous depression
Ulcers
Weak immune system
Wounds

This oil has been used through the ages for various ritual, e.g. as incense in churches. It was one of the gifts brought to baby Jesus by the three wise men. It was also used by the Egyptians as one of the embalming substances. It deepens the breathing, making it a very useful aid in meditation. It is considered to be good for the treatment of ageing skin.

Contra-indications
No known contra-indications. Avoid excessive dosage when first trying this oil.

Experiential note
This oil has a powerful effect on releasing old emotional traumas. Helps to leave them behind, useful when starting something emotionally new in life.

For people who have had a big crisis in life and have lost confidence in themselves or their abilities, blend with jasmine.

IFA compulsory.

GERANIUM

Pelargonium × asperum
Parts used – all parts above ground

Geraniaceae
Note – Middle

Main components
Mono- and sesquiterpenes
Monoterpenols: linalol, alpha-terpineol, citronellol, geraniol, nerol, menthol
Sesquiterpenols
Various esters amounting to 20–30%
Aldehydes: neral, egranial and citronellal
Oxides: cineole
Ketones: methylheptenone,
methone, isomenthone,
piperitone

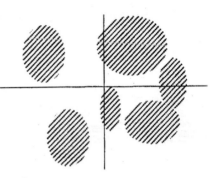

Properties
Antibacterial
Antidepressant
Antifungal
Anti-infectious
Anti-inflammatory
Antiseptic
Antispasmodic
Astringent
Deodorant
Diuretic
General tonic
*Haemostatic
Hepatostimulant
Stimulant for the pancreas
*Tonic for the lymphatic system

Applications
*Cellulite
Colitis of nervous origin
Depression
Dry eczema
Fluid retention
Fungal infections of the skin

Infections of the gums
Itchy piles (especially when combined with *Cupressus sempervirens.*)
Lymphatic drainage (excellent)
Menstrual cycle problems
Neuralgia
Relaxing and antispasmodic to the nervous system
Rheumatism
Shingles
Solar and lower plexus, relaxant as a direct massage of the plexus areas.
Stimulates both the liver and the pancreas
Tonic and astringent for the skin. (Balances sebum secretion)
Varicose and cutaneous ulcers

Contra-indications
As it has an effect on the oestrogen balance it should not be used for persons who have or have had tumorous growths.

Experiential note
Reduces heavy menstrual flows when used during the flow days and the oestrogen phase of the cycle.

IFA compulsory.

GINGER

Zingiber officinale Zingiberaceae
Parts used – roots Note – Top

Main components
Monoterpenes: pinenes, champhene, limonene
Sesquiterpenes (approx. 55%): zinginberene (30%), arcurcumene
Monoterpenols: nerolidol, elemol, zingiberenol
Ketones

Properties
Anticatarrhal
Aphrodisiac
Carminative – relieving
flatulence
Digestive tonic
Expectorant
Stomachich – improving
appetite

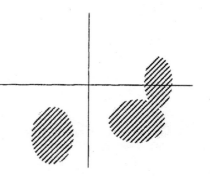

Applications
Catarrh
Chronic bronchitis
Constipation
Dyspepsia
Lack of appetite
Muscular aches and pains
Nervous exhaustion
Poor capillary circulation
Rheumatism
Travel sickness

Contra-indications
No known contra-indications.

Experiential note
A very warming, stimulating oil, rubefacient. The fresh root can be used as a hot infusion to ward off a starting cold. Excellent for all cold, moist conditions.

IFA compulsory.

ITALIAN EVERLASTING

Helichrysum italicum ssp. serotinum

Asteraceae
(Compositae)
Note – Middle

Parts used – flowering tops

Main components
Sesquiterpenes: beta-caryophyllene
Monoterpenols: nerol
Esters: neryl acetate (about 75%)
Ketones: beta-diones

Properties
Anticholesterol
*Anticholesterol
*Antihaematoma
Antiphlebitic
Antispasmodic
Expectorant
Immuno-modulant
Mucolytic
Stimulant of liver function
Wound healing

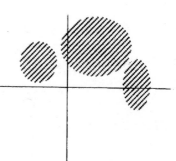

Applications
*Arthritis
Bronchitis
Cholera
*Couperose
*Haematoma external and internal (even old ones)
Headaches of hepatic origin
Herpes
Phlebitis
Polyarthritis
Rhinitis
Spasmodic cough and whooping cough
Viral colitis
Wounds

Contra-indications
Not suitable for subjects that are sensitive to ketones.

Experiential note
Helichrysum italicum is an excellent oil for reducing inflammation and pain in arthritic joints when applied directly to the inflamed areas in normal 2–3% dilutions.

Patricia Davis states that this is a good oil for activating the intuitive right side of the brain, thus this would be useful for therapists or those working with arts and creativity.

JUNIPER

Juniperus communis ssp. communis Cupressaceae
Parts used – berries and twigs Note – Middle

Main components
Mono-terpenes (90%): alpha- and beta-pinenes (40–90% and 1.5–4%), sabinene (10–40%)
Sesquiterpenes: beta-caryophyllene
Sesquiterpenols: alpha-eudesmol, elemol
Esters: bornyl- and terpinenyle acetates
Coumarins: umbelliferone

Properties
Anticatarrhal
*Antiseptic
*Diuretic
Expectorant

Applications
Bronchitis
Cystitis
*Gout
*Rheumatism

Contra-indications

Diuretic oils should not be used continuously. Those with a history of kidney problems should avoid this oil particular as it contains terpene-4-ol.

Juniperus communis var montana

This variety contains more esters which gives it anti-inflammatory and anti-spasmodic action.

Applications

In addition to the above

* *Arthritis*
Inflammatory and spasmodic colitis
* *Sciatica*

Experiential note

Juniper oils are very useful for fluid retention related to the menstrual cycle and also in the treatment of cellulite. It helps clear skin problems such as acne. Purifier at all levels.

IFA compulsory.

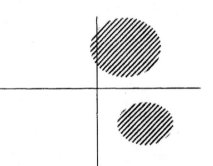

LAVENDER – TRUE

Lavandula angustifolia   Lamiaceae
Also known as *Lavandula vera* or *officinalis*.   (Labiatae)
Parts used – flowering tops   Note – Top

Main components
Alcohols (45%): linalol, lavandulol, terpenol and geraniol
Esters (50%): linalyl acetate, lavandulyl acetate and geranyl acetate
Oxides: cineole
Ketones: camphor

Lavender is sometimes called the mother of essential oils, it has always been considered a general balancer both physically and emotionally. It is a good and safe oil to use for all, including children and babies (if an essential oil is needed for a baby). It is said to have a very strong action on the solar plexus area to calm emotional imbalances and also has been found to be useful for manic depression. It is used on the more esoteric level to cleanse a room or a house from negative influences.

Properties
Analgesic
Anti-infectious
Anti-inflammatory
Antiseptic
Antispasmodic
Bactericide
Calming and sedative
Cicatrisant
Disinfectant
General and heart tonic
Hypotensor
Insecticide
Muscle decongestant
Parasiticide
Regulator of nervous system

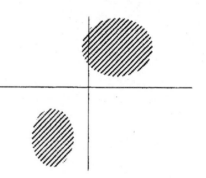

Applications

Acne and acne rosacea
Allergies
Anxiety
Cold and flu especially when a mild and gentle oil is required
Fluctuating moods
Headaches
*Hypertension
*Insomnia and sleep disorders for all ages
*Muscular spasms and congestion especially of the trapezius and solar plexus
Nervous tension
*Night time cramps – for rapid relief, apply neat to the affected area
Palpitations
Scarring
Skin infections
*Stings, bites and burns
*Varicose ulcers – used in combination with tea-tree
Wounds and sores

Contra-indications

No known contra-indications but caution is needed for people who suffer from low blood pressure.

Experiential note

It is necessary for lavender to contain 40–50% esters for it to produce its reputed balancing action or to work as an antispasmodic.

A veritable first aid kit in a bottle.

IFA compulsory.

LAVENDER – SPIKE

Lavandula spica / Lavandula latifolia

Lamiaceae
(Labiatae)

Parts used – shrubs and flowering tops

Note – Top

There are two kinds of spike lavenders on the market; the French and the Spanish. The one that should be used is the French LS, as the Spanish LS is very camphorous which makes it neurotoxic.

Main components of French *Lavandula spica*
Monoterpenes: alpha pinene
Alcohols: linaolol
Oxides: cineole

Properties
Antibacterial
Antifungal
Anti-infectious
Antiviral
Expectorant

Applications
For skin problems, dry acne,
dry eczema, burns, respiratory tract infections even for small children, viral infections in any area.

Contra-indications
No known contra-indications – when no or low camphor composition.

LEMON RINDS

Citrus limon   Rutaceae
Parts used – peel (cold pressed)   Note – Top

Main components
Volatile particles –
Monoterpenes: limonene (54–72%), terpinenes
Sesquiterpenes
Aliphatic alcohols
Aldehydes (2–3%)
Coumarins and furocoumarins:
scopoletine, umbelliferone,
bergamottine, bergaptole,
bergaptene
Non-volatile particles
(approx 2%): flavonoides,
carotenoides, steroids

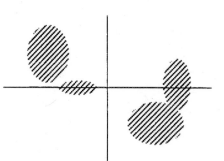

Properties
Anti-infectious (bacteria,
parasites, viruses)
Antiseptic
Calming of the nervous system
Carminative
Litholytic

Applications
Cellulitis
Gout
Insomnia
Insufficient liver, pancreas, gallbladder functions
Kidney- and gallstones
Oily skin

Phlebitis
Poor circulation
Respiratory infections
*Rheumatism
Thrombosis
*Varicose vein
Warts

Some of the coumarins in this oil have an anticoagulant property.

This oil is particular effective as an air antiseptic during periods of contagious diseases.

Contra-indications
Photosensitizing. Skin irritant due to the citrals. Be aware of deterpenated lemon oil; it will have an increased action of the citrals. Skin irritation can also be caused by the residues of the sprays used during the growing, which are transferred into the essence during the extraction.

Experiential note
An excellent oil for easing the discomforts of and reducing varicose veins.

Try this experiment on the effect of lemon oil on the digestion system (this arose from a reported Japanese study on lemon oil).

> Think of a lemon. See it clearly, its shape and colour. Imagine that you scratch the skin and smell the spray. Then cut the lemon in half and smell its aroma. What is happening to you now?
>
> Yes, you are salivating and you did not even smell the lemon.
>
> The result of the Japanese study is reputed to be that smelling the essential oil of lemon is more effective in easing digestive problems than taking the oil internally. You have just proved to yourself the increased salivation! The body's own enzymes in the saliva are the most effective aids for digestion.

Suitable for the sanguine temperament.

IFA compulsory.

MANDARIN

Citrus reticulata　　　　　　　　　　　　　　　　Rutaceae
Parts used – peel (cold pressed)　　　　　　　　　Note – Top

Main components
Volatile particles –
Monoterpenes (<94%): limonene
Non-terpenic alcohols: nonanol, oxtanol
Monoterpenols: citronellol, linalol
Esters
Aldehydes
Coumarins and furocoumarins

This oil has some non-volatile
particles

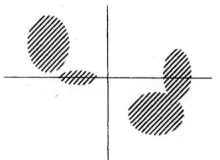

Properties
Antifungal
Antiseptic activity
Antispasmodic
Balances central nervous
system
Digestive tonic (helps digestion in the stomach)
Helps in the production of bile
Hypnotic
*Relaxant
*Sedative

Applications
Digestive system problems of nervous origin
Dyspepsia and hiccoughs
Excitability
*Insomnia

Contra-indications

This oil is not suitable to use before sunbathing or sunlamp use as it makes the skin photosensitive.

No other contra-indications are known.

Skin irritation can also be caused by the residues of the sprays used during the growing, which are transferred into the essence during the extraction.

Experiential note

This oil is useful for people suffering from sleep disorders related to digestive problems.

IFA compulsory.

MARJORAM – SWEET

Origanum majorana   Lamiaceae
                                                      (Labiatae)
Parts used – flowering heads/leaves   Note – Middle

Main components
Monoterpenes (40%): pinenes, sabinene, terpinenes, paracymene
Sesquiterpenes: beta caryophyllene
Monoterpenols (about 50%): linalol, terpinene-4-ol, alpha-terpineol, thujanol-4
Esters: terpenyl acetate, linalyl acetate, geranyl acetate

Properties
Analgesic
Anaphrodisiac
Antibacterial
Anti-infectious
Antiseptic
Diuretic
Hypotensive
Neurotonic
Stimulates the parasympathetic
nervous system
Vaso-dilator

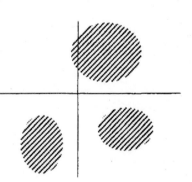

Applications
*Anxiety
Asthenia
Bronchitis
Coughs
Diarrhoea
Enterocolitis
*Grief
*Hypertension
Hyperthyroid conditions
*Insomnia
*Muscle aches and sprains
Neuralgia
Otitis
*Painful joints
*Rheumatic pain
Sinusitis
Tachycardia
Vertigo
Whooping cough

Contra-indications
No known contra-indications in normal doses.

Experiential note
Very warming and comforting oil for all stress-related conditions.

Using this oil in combination with *Boswellia carterii* boosts the effectiveness of each oil in releasing old holds from tissue memory, and assists in clearing them.

NOT TO BE USED

<u>GREAT MUGWORT</u>

Artemisia arborescence   Asteraceae
                                                         (Compositae)

Parts used – leaves and flowering tops   Note

Main components
Monoterpenes: limonene, sabinene
Sesquiterpenes: chamazulene, dihyrochamazulene
Oxides: epoxycaryophylene
Monoterpenones: isothujone
(30–40%) camphor (23–18%)

Properties
Anti-allergic
Anticatarrhal
Antihistaminic
Anti-inflammatory
Mucolytic

Applications
Asthma
Catarrhal and asthmatic bronchitis
Insufficient secretion of bile

Contra-indications
Babies
Young children
Pregnant women (neurotoxic and abortive)

This oil is sometimes sold as *Matricaria recutita* and is only included here to enable comparison between them.

MYRRH

Commiphora molmol
Parts used – oleo resin

Burseraceae
Note – Top

Main components
Sesquiterpenes: elemenes (about 29%), alpha copaene (about 10%)
Furanic sesquiterpenes: curzerene
Furanic sesquiterpenone: curzerenone
Ketones: methyl-isobutyl ketone (about 5%)
Aldehydes: 3 methyl-1, 2-butenal

Properties
Anaphrodisiac
Anti-infectious
Anti-inflammatory
Antiviral
Moderator of thyroid action
Parasiticide

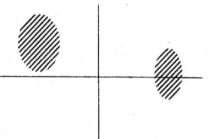

Applications
Bronchitis
Diarrhoea
Dysentery
Hyperthyroidism
*Mouth ulcers
Viral hepatitis

Contra-indications
Pregnant women

Experiential note
Myrrh oil diluted in alcohol is very useful as one option for *athletes foot*.

Has similar action to *Boswellia carterii* in releasing old emotions, often in dreams.

NEROLI BIGARADE
(Orange Flower)

Citrus aurantium ssp. aurantium   Rutaceae
Parts used – flowers   Note – Top

Main components
Monoterpenes (35%): pinenes, limonene
Monoterpenols (40%): linalol, alpha-terpineol, geraniol, nerol
Sesquiterpenols: trans-nerolidol, farnesol
Esters: linalyl acetate, neryl acetate, geranyl acetate
Aldehydes: decanal, benzal
Ketones: jasmone

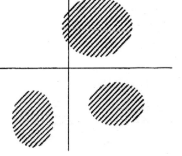

Properties
Antibacterial
Antidepressant
Anti-infectious
Antiparasitic
Cellular regenerator
Digestive tonic
(hepatopancreatic)
Hypotensive
Neurotonic (recharges and balances)

Applications
Arterial hypertension
Bacterial and parasitic enterocolitis
Bronchitis
Fatigue
Haemorrhoids
Nervous depression
Pleurisy
Stimulates liver and pancreas functions
Tuberculosis
Varicose veins

Contra-indications
No known contra-indications.

Experiential note
This is undoubtedly one of the very best anti-stress oils. It helps to relax both the mind and the body and allows the mind to take a holiday from constant racing and chatter. Yet it does not make one feel drowsy but gives energy and helps to find new approaches to deal with problems.

IFA compulsory.

NIAOULI

Melaleuca quinquenervia – viridiflorol   Myrtaceae
Parts used – leaves   Note – Top

Main components
Monoterpenes: pinenes, limonene
Sesquiterpenes: beta-caryophyllene, viridiflorene
Monoterpenols: linalol, terpene-4-ol, alpha-terpineol
Sesquiterpenols: globulol, viridiflorol
Aldehydes: isovaleraldehyde, benzaldehyde
Oxides: cineole

Properties
Antibacterial
Anticatarrhal
Anti-infectious
Anti-inflammatory
Antiparasitic
Antiviral
Antiseptic
Decongestant of veins
Expectorant
Helps control high blood pressure
Oestrogen like
Skin tonic
Useful for allergic reactions

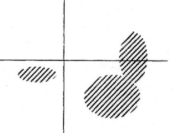

Applications
Arterio-sclerosis
Boils
Bronchitis
Catarrh
Cholera
Diarrhoea
Gastric and duodenal ulcers
Haemorrhoids
Herpes
Nervous depression, especially due to viral infections
Psoriasis

Rheumatoid arthritis
Sinusitis
Sluggish liver functions
Tonsillitis
Tuberculosis
*Varicose veins
Viral enteritis
Vulvovaginitis

Contra-indications
No known contra-indications, but young children should be careful with this oil.

Experiential note
Young people and teenagers find this oil very useful for acne and boils, especially since it also works through the hormonal system. I use this oil often in a blend for haemorrhoids and varicose veins. This is also an excellent oil for imbalances in the menstrual cycle.

PALMAROSA – INDIAN

Cymbopogon martinii – var. motia

Poaceae
(Graminaceae)
Note – Top

Parts used – whole plant

Main components
Monoterpenols (80–95%): linalol, geraniol (70–80%), nerol
Sesquiterpenols: elemol
Esters: geranyl acetate, geranyl- and neryl formiates

Properties
*Antibacterial with a broad spectrum of action
Antifungal
Antimicrobial
Antiviral
Heart tonic
Nerve tonic
Uterine tonic

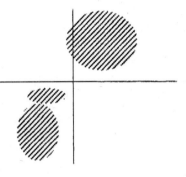

Applications
*Acne
Bacterial and viral enteritis
Bronchitis
Childbirth
Cystitis
*Eczema
Otitis
Sinusitis
Vaginitis

Contra-indications
No known contra-indications – no acute toxicity.

Experiential note
Supports the nervous system – useful for MS. Good results in psoriasis treatment when blended with evening primrose oil or others which have a high GLA content.

One of the few oils that can be introduced into the childbirth situation to support mother and not cause baby to be drowsy.

Both my students and I have used this oil to treat multiple sclerosis sufferers – it supports the nervous system and has a tonifying action.

PEPPERMINT

Mentha × piperita

Lamiaceae
(Labiatae)

Parts used – flowering tops

Note – Top

Mints are native to Europe. Now there are many cultivated hybrids which have become naturalised. Throughout history mints have been used to relieve digestive problems. They are also very useful for colds and flu, especially for the upper respiratory area. Mints are described as cephalic as they can help physically to clear the head, therefore, they may assist thinking processes by stimulating the activity of the brain.

Main components

Monoterpenes: alpha- and beta-pinene
Monoterpenols: menthol and piperitol
Oxides: cineole, piperitonoxide
Ketones: menthone, piperitone
Esters: menthyl acetate

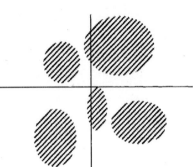

Properties

Analgesic
Antibacterial
Anticatarrhal and expectorant
Anti-infectious, general
Antiviral
Carminative
Digestive stimulant
Fungicide
General tonic and stimulant
Hypertensive
Mucolytic
Secretolytic menthol
Tonic

Applications
*Asthenia
Colitis
Cystitis
Dysmenorrhoea
*Dyspepsia
Eczema
Halitosis
*Indigestion
Inflammatory colitis
Laryngitis
*Migraines and headaches
*Neuralgia
Otitis
Prostatitis
*Sciatica
Sinusitis
Travel sickness
Urticaria

Contra-indications
Not suitable to be used simultaneously with homoeopathic remedies. Not to be used for long periods continuously. Not to be used for children under 3 years of age.

Experiential note
A good oil for shingles when combines with *Chamaemelum nobile*, or *Pelargonium × asperum*.

This is also a good oil to use as an insect repellent.

Definitely a day-time stimulating oil, not to be used late afternoon or evening. Peppermint is also one of the most powerful analgesic oils and is wonderful for headaches and sciatica.

IFA compulsory.

PETITGRAIN
(Orange Leaf)

Citrus aurantium ssp. aurantium Rutaceae
Parts used – leaves Note – Top

Main components
Monoterpenes: myrcene
Monoterpenols (40%): linalol, alpha-terpineol, nerol, geraniol
Esters (50%): linalyl acetate, neryl acetate, terpenyl acetate, geranyl acetate

Properties
Anti-infectious
Anti-inflammatory
Antispasmodic
*Calming and balances the
nervous system*

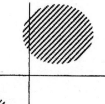

Applications
Acne
Asthma of nervous origin
Osteoarthritis, juvenile
rheumatism, which is of
nervous origin
Respiratory tract infections

Contra-indications
No known contra-indications.

Experiential note
This oil is useful for depression and stress, especially combined with *Citrus aurantium ssp. bergamia*.

Pine – Scotch

Pinus sylvestris

Abietaceae
(Pinaceae)

Parts used – needles and new cones

Note – Middle

Main components
Monoterpenes: (up to 80%), alpha- and beta-pinenes, limonene
Sesquiterpenes: longifolene
Monoterpinols: borneol
Sesquiterpinols: alpha-cadinol
Esters: bornyl acetate

Properties
Antidiabetic
Antifungal
Anti-infectious
*Antiseptic
*Cortisone-like
Decongestant of lymphatic
system
Hormone-like
Hypertensive
Neurotonic
*Sexual and general stimulant
Tonic

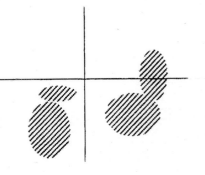

Applications
Arthritis
*Asthenia
Asthma
*Bronchitis
Diabetes
*Inflammatory and allergic reactions
Rheumatoid polyarthritis
Sinusitis
Uterine congestion

Contra-indications
No known contra-indications.

Experiential note
Very stimulating masculine oil for depleted energy at all levels. Clearing of old feelings of guilt, cleansing of the whole system.

In Finland many of the hospitals that deal particularly with respiratory problems are situated in areas of strong pines. Also the newest dermatology and allergy hospitals are placed in the cleansing and healing vicinity of pines.

Prof. R. Hiltunen compared the air composition taken near a pine tree to the essential oil of the same pine tree and found that both samples contained the same particles.

RAVENSARA

Ravensara aromatica   Lauraceae
Parts used – leaves   Note – Middle/top

Main components
Monoterpenes: alpha- and beta-pinene
Sesquiterpenes: betacaryophyllene
Monoterpenols
Esters: terpenyl acetate
Oxides: cineole

Properties
Antibacterial
Expectorant
Neurotonic
Powerful antiviral
Soporific, suits a nervous
temperament
Very positive oil

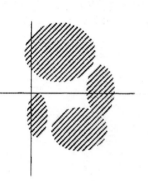

Applications
Asthma
Bronchitis
Chicken pox
Insomnia
Herpes simplex
Herpes zoster
Influenza (excellent)
Muscular fatigue
Sinusitis
Viral enteritis
Whooping cough

The skin tolerance of this oil is excellent.

Contra-indications
No known contra-indications.

Experiential note
Excellent for asthmatic conditions. No cases of adverse reactions to this oil have come to my knowledge.

ROSEMARY

Rosmarinus pyramidalis

Lamiaceae
(Labiatae)

Parts used – leaves and flowering tops

Note – Middle

Main components
Monoterpenes: alpha- and beta-pinene
Monoterpenols: borneol
Oxides: cineole, (the major component of this particular CT)
Monoterpenones: camphor

Properties
Anticatarrhal
Anti-infectious
Cephalic
Expectorant
Mucolytic

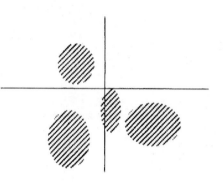

Applications
Bronchitis
Fainting
*General debility
*Hair care
*Hypotension
*Muscular pain and spasm
Otitis
*Physical and mental strain
Sinusitis
Vertigo

Rosemary is as old in its medicinal uses as lavender. Generally stimulating in its effect on the central nervous system and the brain. It assists in lowering cholesterol levels in the blood. Traditionally used for rheumatism, arthritis and hair care. Rosemary stimulates the adrenal cortex and raises blood pressure.

Contra-indications
Epilepsy
High blood pressure

Experiential note
Pyramidalis type of rosemary generally has the lowest ketone content, as compared with other types of rosemary, and therefore has a lesser possibility of causing irritation.

Helps to maintain concentration when having to do mental work continuously for long periods.

IFA compulsory.

ROSEWOOD – BOIS DE ROSE

Aniba rosaeodora   Lauraceae
Parts used – wood   Note – Top

Main components
Monoterpenols: linalol (95%)

Properties
Antibacterial
Antifungal
Anti-infectious
Antiparasitic
Antiviral
General tonic and stimulant
Very positive oil due to its
large alcohol content

Applications
Asthenia
Bronchial problems for all ages, including babies
Calming of nervousness, but refreshing
Candidal infections of the vagina
Depression of the nervous type
Ear, nose and throat infections

This oil is gentle in its actions in all areas. It is useful for headaches, especially if the headache is associated with nausea. It clarifies thinking and therefore is a useful oil for exams and any kind of stress or crisis situations.

Contra-indications
No known contra-indications.

Experiential note
This oil has an ability to strengthen emotionally and to centre one in himself. It seems to have an ability to dispel fear and I feel it is especially good for nervous people or those that are afraid to face themselves. This oil is *particularly pleasant and suitable for the elderly.*

Some students have found that rosewood is a good mosquito repellent.

Controversy over the use of this oil has risen because of the destruction of the rain forests after the building of the roads to the rosewood areas. Ho-wood oil has been suggested as a replacement. I have no experience of hoewood, but as it contains a fair amount of ketones it is not suitable as a substitute. Try *Thymus vulgaris ct. linaloliferum* instead.

SANDALWOOD

Santalum album   Santalaceae
Parts used – roots and wood   Note – Base

Main components
Sesquiterpenes: santalenes
Sesquiterpenols: santalols (67%)
Aldehydes: teresantalal

Properties
Antiseptic in the urinary tract
Calming and soothing
Cardiotonic
Lymphatic and venous
decongestant

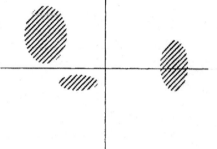

Applications
Cardiac fatigue
Cystitis
*Depression
Haemorrhoids
Insomnia
*Lumbago
Neuralgia
Respiratory infections
*Sciatica
*Skin care for dry, chapped, and oily skin
Varicose veins

Contra-indications
No known contra-indications.
Can cause digestive problems and kidney irritation.

Traditionally used as an incense to clear negative influences.

Experimental note
A powerful aphrodisiac especially if combined with *Cananga odorata*.

SPRUCE – BLACK

Picea mariana

Abietaceae
(Pinaceae)

Parts used – needles

Note – Top – Middle

Main components
Monoterpenes: camphene, tricyclene, alpha-pinene, carene
Sesquiterpenes: longifolene, longicyclene
Monoterpenols: borneol
Sesquiterpenols: longiborneol
Esters: bornyl acetate

Properties
Anti-infectious
Anti-inflammatory
Antiparasitic
Antispasmodic
Cortisone-like
General and neurotonic and
a recharger
Very stimulating, positive oil

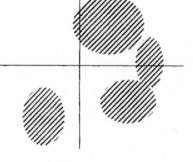

Applications
Acne
Adrenal insufficiency
Asthenia
Bronchitis
Candidal inflammation of the mucosa of the small intestine
Dry eczema
Hyperthyroid conditions
Inflamed, painful, damaged joints
Inflammatory prostatitis
Muscular rheumatism
Solar plexus spasm
Sprained joints and ligaments

Generally a very stimulating, very tonifying masculine oil. No acute toxicity.

Contra-indications
No known contra-indications, but can irritate the skin if used for more than 3–5 days continuously in high dosages.

Experiential note
Picea mariana makes a very stimulating recharging blend for exhaustion with *Pinus sylvestris* and *Pelargonium* × *asperum* when one needs to keep going for a day or two. Not advisable for continuous use.

For cheering and recharging; *Picea mariana* and *Citrus paradisi* or *Citrus aurantium bergamia* make a delicious, delightful blend. For inflamed damaged joints a cold compress of *Picea mariana* and *Eucalyptus citriodora* brings rapid relief.

TARRAGON

Artemisia dracunculus

Asteraceae
(Compositae)

Part used – flowering plant

Note – Top

Main components
Phenol-monomethyl-ethers: chavicol ME (60–75%)
Coumarins

Properties
Anti-allergic
Anti-infectious
Anti-inflammatory
Antispasmodic of the
neuromuscular system
Antiviral
Very positive oil

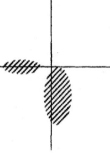

Applications
Deficiency of kidney function
*Dysmenorrhoea
*Muscular spasms
Nervous fatigue
Neuralgia
*Sciatica
Spasmodic and inflammatory colitis
Tetanus

Contra-indications
No known contra-indications.

Experiential note
Blended with *Mentha × piperita* and *Betula alleghaniensis* this oil makes an excellent blend for muscles that are painful and aching due to hard spasm from overuse.

<u>TEA-TREE</u>

Melaleuca alternifolia   Myrtaceae
Parts used – leaves   Note – Top

This is a shrub that favours wet grounds. It grows up to 5 metres in height, it has paper like bark (it is called paper bark by the natives) and leaves that are no more than 2 centimetres long and almost needle like in their shape. Traditionally in Australia the tea-tree oil is used for infected fingernail beds, cuts from corals, boils, mouth ulcers, general cuts and abrasions, pyorrhoea and gonorrhoea. It was also used widely during the second World War as a general germicidal and healing agent.

Main components
Monoterpenes: pinenes, myrcene, terpinenes, paracymene, limonene, terpinolene
Sesquiterpenes: beta caryophyllene, aromadendrene, viridiflorene
Monoterpenols: terpinene 4-ol, alpha-terpineol
Sesquiterpenols: globulol, viriflorol
Oxides: cineole

Properties
Antifungal
Anti-infectious
Antiparasitic
Antiviral
Broad spectrum of direct antibacterial action
Cardiotonic
Cicatrisant
Decongestant of veins
Generally stimulating and positive oil
Immunostimulant
Neurotonic

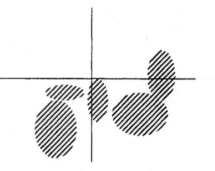

Applications
Asthenia
Enterocolitis; bacterial, candidal, viral and parasitic
General debility
General depression, indicating multiple functional deficiencies
in the immune system

Genital infections
Gingivitis
Haemorrhoids and varicose veins
Nervous depression, especially in nervous types
Lack of general physical tone
*Preventative of post-operative shock related to the anaesthetic
Respiratory pathways
Slowed capillary circulation
Tooth abscesses

This oil is especially well known for its efficiency against candida albicans and the problems related to it, providing it contains a min. 25% terpinene-4-ol.

Recommended for people who have constant recurring infections and also those who need to use antibiotics to boost the immune system.

Contra-indications
Terpinene-4-ol is a kidney irritant, therefore this oil should not be used for persons with impaired kidney function or suffering from kidney infections.

Experiential note
Excellent experiences in recovery both mentally and physically from operations when using this oil prior to surgery. This oil has also excellent cicatrisant properties.

Melaleuca alternifolia could be said to be almost as good a First Aid in a bottle as *Lavandula angustifolia*.

IFA compulsory.

THYME – COMMON

Thymus vulgaris – ct. linaloliferum   Lamiaceae
                                                        (Labiatae)

Parts used – flowers and leaves   Note – Top to middle

Main components
Monoterpenes
Monoterpenols: linalol (60-80%)
Esters: linalyl acetate

Properties
Antibacterial
Antimicrobial
Antiparasitic
Antispasmodic
Antiviral
*Fungicide, especially for
candida albicans*
General tonic and neurotonic
Tonic for uterus, also
considered an aphrodisiac
Very positive oil

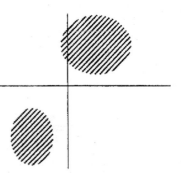

Applications
Bronchial pneumonia
Bronchitis
Candidal infection of vagina
Muscular rheumatism
Nervous fatigue
Pleurisy
Psoriasis

Contra-indications
No known contra-indications.

YARROW

Achillea liqustica
Parts used – leaves and flowering tops

Asteraceae
Note – not known

Main components
Sesquiterpenes: chamazulene, dihyroazulenes
Monoterpenones: camphor and thujones
Oxides: cineole

Properties
Anticatarrhal
Anti-infectious
Anti-inflammatory
Antispasmodic
Astringent
Choleretic
Cicatrisant
Laxative
Emmenagogue
Immunostimulant

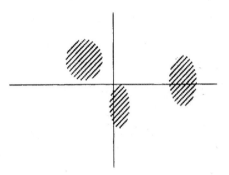

Applications
Constipation
Digestive stimulant
Dysmenorrhoea
Gastristis
Haemorrhoids
Inflammatory entercolitis
Neuritis and neuralgia
Respiratory catarrhal infections
Rheumatism
Wounds

Contra-indications
Babies
Young children
Pregnant women

Neurotoxic and abortive. Acute toxicity due to ketones.

YLANG YLANG/FLOWER OF FLOWERS

Cananga odorata forma genuina   Anonaceae
Parts used – flowers   Note – Middle

Main components
Sesquiterpenes: alpha-farnesene
Alcohols, monoterpenic and aromatic: linalol 55%, benzylic alcohol
Sesquiterpenols: farnesol
Esters: geranyl and benzyl acetate, 5% and 10%, benzyl benzoate
Phenol-methyl-ethers: p-cresol M.E. 15%

Properties
Antispasmodic
Emotional balancer
Sexual tonic

Applications
Frigidity
Hypertension
Tachycardia – anxiety, rapid
breath, panic

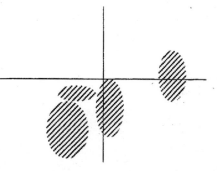

Ylang ylang has been called the poor man's Jasmine, possibly because of its flower aroma. It is widely used in perfumery and skin care.

Contra-indications
No known contra-indications, but this oil clearly has an effect on reducing blood pressure.

Experiential note
Cananga odorata is an excellent aid in menopausal problems. Using it as a daily treatment of two drops to the abdomen and lower back will clear 'hot flushes' and help to reduce the dryness of the mucous membranes.

Students both in Finland and England have found this oil excellent in relieving the discomfort of Crohns disease. As yet I have not found a definite reason for this, but a clue may be in its beneficial effect on the mucous membranes, as in Crohns disease the lining of the bowel loses its protective mucous and elasticity, and also as it relieves the colicky pains caused by Crohns.

IFA compulsory.

ESSENTIAL OILS THAT ARE PARTICULARLY GOOD FOR EMOTIONAL CONDITIONS

For emotional conditions the dosage of the essential oils can be very low – one or two drops inhaled is usually enough.

Angelica archangelica, Angelica

This is a very good oil to relieve unexplained anxiety that arises from the personality. Angelica is also a good oil for insomnia.

Aniba rosaeodora, Rosewood

Helpful in stressful situations where calmness and clarity of the mind are required, also for the nervous temperament that is afraid to express and be oneself.

Boswellia carterii, Frankincense

Cananga odorata, Ylang ylang

An excellent oil for frustrated anger, particularly if combined with *Chamaemelum nobile*. This essential oil eases anxiety and fears with unknown causes.

Chamaemelum nobile, Roman Chamomile

Half a drop is enough for children's temper tantrums and sleep disorders. For adults this oil relieves situations where an angry response would bring relief, but the situation makes it an inappropriate reaction. A calming and soothing oil that is also useful in cleansing away old emotional aches and fears. Avoid excessive dosages – effect will be reversed.

Citrus aurantium ssp. bergamia, Bergamot

For excessive mood swings particularly for the young, e.g. teenagers, and also for premenstrual moodiness.

Note this oil is photosensitizing, so use it in a vaporiser or lamp, not on the skin.

An interesting find of this oil is that though generally very uplifting in its effect, when burned it tends to make people under the influence of alcohol tearful and sad.

Citrus aurantium ssp. aurantium, Neroli bigarade orange flowers

This is especially good for stressful conditions, when rest is not possible, as this oil gives clarity to the situation and refreshes both mind and body.

Citrus paradisi, Grapefruit

Grapefruit essential oil is a real joy. Inhaled it will uplift the mind and banish tiredness. A Spring cleaning of the mind!

Note this oil is photosensitizing, so use it in a vaporiser or lamp, not on the skin.

Citrus reticulata, Mandarin

For depression that causes insomnia, anxiety and irritability.

Note this oil is photosensitizing, so use it in a vaporiser or lamp, not on the skin.

Jasminum officinale, Jasmine

This is a confidence booster. A very powerful oil for those who have been through a burnout or who, through some other disappointment have lost their trust in life and belief in themselves. Jasmine is also the oil that terminally ill people tend to choose for themselves. Adding *Boswellia carterii* (Frankincense) to Jasmine helps to let go of life and old holds when coming to the end of life.

On long journeys, Jasmine has a very good ability, when combined with Neroli, to lift tiredness from driving.

Melissa officinalis, Melissa

This is an excellent essential oil that is difficult to find in its true undiluted, unadulterated form, but if found it is a real treasure to banish the dooms and glooms. It is difficult to find words that describe the feeling of light, brightness and alert awareness that it gives when inhaled. *Lippia citriodora* is a rarity in the essential oils and its effects are as powerful as those melissa gives, though the feeling is more green and euphoric, and not as clear.

Rosa damascena, Rose

One drop of true rose oil is enough to lift a depression. It really does warm the heart and ease its sorrows and pain. True rose will even coax an expression of joy from those that are so ill that they have very little ability to respond consciously. It is a flower of compassion, devotion and love and when accompanied with these emotions from the therapist, have a very deep healing ability.

Santalum album, Sandalwood

Sandalwood has always been used in India, its country of origin, as a spiritual oil, to help in meditation and to clear negativity. This is an oil for the emotional area of the body and assists in strengthening and grounding emotions.

Vetiveria zizanoides, Vetiver
This oil has a powerful calming effect on the mind. It also appears to have the ability to root ones feet into the ground and emotions to realities in a very positive strengthening way. Its initially smoky aroma may at first be a shock, but on skin it changes to a pleasant, very sweet, woody moss odour.

CONTRA-INDICATIONS
There are not many general contra-indications to the use of the essential oils, but more to the massage part of aromatherapy. These are indicated by the letters **M** for NO massage and **E** for NO essential oil.

Alcohol, Drugs	M	E	All essential oils alter the effect of alcohol
Babies	M	E	No massage for under six weeks
Cancer, chemotherapy	M	E	Except for terminal cases
Enlarged lymph noted	M		
Fever	M		
Fluid retention	M	E	If due to heart or kidney problems
Haemophilia	M		
Infectious Disease	M		
Injuries, new			
– sprains, pulls	M		
– wound, bruises	M		
Ischaemia	M		Avoid powerfully stimulating oils
Leg ulcers	M		
Medication, acute or long term	M		Check with doctor
Operations	M		Depending on the severity check with surgeon
Pregnancy, breast feeding		E	
Serious illnesses	M	E	Consult with GP
Shock	M		
Skin conditions			
• allergy	M		Check for allergy to essential oil
• boil	M		
• cuts / grazes	M		
• infection	M		
• psoriasis	M		
Vaccinations	M		No massage for 7 days
Varicose veins /venous congestion	M		

If not certain, no treatment

4 Vegetable Carrier Oils and Hydrolats

VEGETABLE CARRIER OILS

Use cold pressed wherever possible, as deodorising and other processing will rob the oils of nutritional and healing properties.

When using nut oils check for allergies.

Almond Oil (Sweet)
> Pale yellow, fairly thick, easy to massage with. Good for most skin types and suited to body massage blends. Contains vitamins and minerals. Strengthens nails.

Apricot Kernel
> Light texture and pale colour. Suitable for facial massage blends and therapeutic massage. Good for mature, sensitive and dry skins – easily absorbed into the skin.

Avocado (refined)
> Excellent for facial massage blends – one of the heaviest oils, useful for treating mature skin. Contains protein, vitamins, lecithin and essential fatty acids, easily absorbed, carrying its nutritional vitamins and essential fatty acids into the deeper levels of the skin. Blocks out the sun's rays and protects the skin.

Borage Oil
> Rich in vitamins, minerals and GLA. Good to treat psoriasis. Borage is reputed to have a beneficial effect on the mind and body. May cause irritation, warming when first applied to the skin.

Calendula – maceration
> Marigolds macerated, usually in sunflower or olive oil. Softening and soothing for skin, e.g. cracked or dry feet. Calendula has a reputation for healing all types of skin problems.

Camellia

Light non-greasy texture. Rich in healing nutritive elements for nervous tissue of skin. Quickly absorbed, perfect for facial massage and skin-care blends.

Carrot – maceration

A maceration in sunflower. Rich in carotenes and a good source of vitamins. Anti-ageing. Anti-free radicals. Useful for helping tanning.

Evening Primrose

Sticky and heavy in texture. The gamma linoleic acid will be absorbed into the upper layers of the skin and help prevent loss of moisture. A good oil to use for many skin problems. Especially beneficial for psoriasis and eczema used internally and externally.

Grape Seed

Light texture and has no smell. Many therapists find it good for body massage. Suits all skin types. Cannot be cold pressed.

Hazelnut

Easily absorbed, suits oily or combination skins. Good for face and body massage. Rich in vitamin E making it a natural anti-oxidant.

Jojoba (Dis.Deo.)

Excellent for daily skin care, for cleansing and protecting. Oil extracted from the bean. Wax-like; colourless and odourless. Excellent base for facial blends. Fine texture, good skin penetration – too dry for body massage. Semi-wax-like; rich in vitamin E. Composition close to skin's own sebum. Contains natural anti-bacterial properties which give it fairly lasting life before turning rancid. Excellent for protection from sun and cold.

Macadamia Nut

Rich in texture. Useful in remedial purposes where blood pressure and cholesterol levels are a factor. Virgin, cold pressed. It has a notice-able aroma. A good oil in blends of carriers.

Rose Hip (Muscat) winterized

Healing, regenerating. Useful for scars, skin burns, premature ageing. Not good for oily or acne skin conditions.

Sesame Seed
> For those who are allergic to nut oils, rich texture and a sesame aroma. Natural moisturizer, gives some sun protection.

St. John's Wort – maceration
> In virgin, cold pressed olive oil. This red oil has remarkable skin soothing and healing properties. Anti-inflammatory. Useful for sciatica etc. Soothing for irritated and inflamed skin, psoriasis etc. Care needs to be taken not to be used in direct sunlight – photo-sensitizing. Excellent as a base for sciatica blend.

Walnut
> Virgin, cold pressed. Good for all-round massage. High in un-saturated fatty acids, particularly GLA. Makes the skin feel very soft and satin like.

Wheatgerm
> Cold pressed. A rich yellow colour with a distinct wheaten aroma. Excellent source of vitamin E, good for healing scar tissue and burns. Natural anti-oxidant. Rich in nutritives, for dry and mature skin.

HYDROLATS – FLOWER WATERS

These are by-products of the distillation process. The most water soluble aromatic molecules from the plant delicately fragrance the distillation water, so that there is a 'shadow' of the essential oil. Use is general for swabbing wounds, rashes, baby's skin, and as compresses and poultices. They are very good used as skin toners, as they are alcohol free. Useful for all age groups and skin types.

Chamaemelum nobile
For infected and inflamed skin, compresses for tired, sore eyes or eye infections. Babies' skin irritations.

Helichrysum italicum
Bruised tissue, open skin, abscesses, couperoses. Sedative.

Juniperus communis
Astringent for acne and oily skin. Refreshing.

Lavandula angustifolia
All skin types and all problems. Balancing. Excellent for burnt, stinging skin, soothing it very rapidly.

Melissa officinalis
Calming for irritated skins. Sedative.

Rosa damascena
Couperoses, wrinkled skin, dermatitis. Broken and sensitive skins. Sedative.

Thymus vulgaris – Thujanol 4
Sluggish circulation, dull and lifeless skin. Energising.

Laurus nobilis
Greasy skin, skin infections, acne.

5 *Aromatherapy Massage*

THE HISTORY OF MASSAGE

The roots of massage are found at the very beginning of human history. It is possibly the oldest method of healing. We all know stroking a hurt is an instinctive reaction, and a mother naturally and automatically will stroke a child's hurt. The oldest written records are from China (2700 BC) where massage is regarded as the oldest medicinal method together with acupuncture and medicinal herbs. The ayurvedic medicine records from 1800 BC mention massage. Also the Egyptian, Persian and Japanese historical records indicate it as a form of medical treatment. Ancient Greeks used massage at all levels of society, after baths, for pleasure, after illness for speedy recovery, before athletic effort to warm the tissues and protect them from damage and after the effort to recover the tone of the muscles and to relieve pain. It seems that massages were given not only by the medical practitioners, but also by priests and slaves. There was also a professional body of masseurs whose job it was to oil the wrestler both before and after the competition.

Herodikus one of **Hippocrates'** teachers appeared to be the first to use exercises and massage as specific forms of treatment. Hippocrates himself (460–377 BC) was so proficient in massage as to be able to name illnesses for which massage was a beneficial method of treatment and also those illnesses that he felt that massage was not suited. He especially recommended massage for dislocated joints and sprains. In his opinion a physician must be proficient in many things, but especially in massage. Though the circulatory system was not known, Hippocrates found that upward, towards-the-heart directed massage of the limbs gave better results than a downward massage.

Swedish teacher of fencing **P.E. Ling** (1776–1839) became an authority on massage having cured rheumatism in his own arms with massage. According to Ling, massage is like passive exercising. He based his system on the then new science of physiology. This method became known as the Ling method of Swedish Movement Therapy. In 1813, at the Stockholm's Kungliga

Gymnastike Institute, massage was accepted as an official subject of study. The Ling method became known throughout the world and training institutes were established. It was not until 1899 when Sir William Bennett included massage treatment at St. George's Hospital that interest in massage was awakened in England.

In 1952, American **Gertrude Bear** defined massage as follows:

"Massage is a term which is used to describe certain kinds of soft tissue manipulation which is aimed to have an effect on the nervous, muscular and respiratory systems. Also increases local or general blood and lymph circulation."

MASSAGE STROKES

The Classical or Swedish massage strokes are divided into five main groups; effleurage, friction, petrissage/kneading, tapotage and vibration. Although the strokes are divided into these basic sets of movements the performance of them differs and varies according to the part of the body massaged and also the aim of the treatment.

Effleurage

In effleurage the hand, or part of the hand, glides across the skin moulding completely to the tissues under it. Especially on the limbs the movement is directed towards the centre of the body, in other words following the venous circulation. The movement is begun lightly, increasing pressure towards to the centre of the muscle and lightly again towards the end, before coming off the skin. The lighter the effleurage stroke is the more it affects the surface tissues. The deeper and stronger the movement the deeper the tissues are affected. Both of these types of effleurage can be performed as long or short movements depending on the required effect. Effleurage can be performed with the whole hand, the palm, the base of the hand or with thumbs or fingers depending on the size of the area to be treated and how deep the stroke is aimed. The effleurage movement can be performed with just one hand or both hands together or alternating the two hands, one starting when the other one is beginning to lift. It is in this alternating hand movement that you have to be particularly aware of the rhythm of the strokes. Effleurage is as a rule, used at the beginning of the treatment, but also as a connecting move between different strokes or the different areas of the body. It is with the effleurage movement that the patient becomes familiar with the touch of the therapist.

This is one of the reasons why they need to be performed rhythmically but very calmly. During the effleurage movements the therapist begins to sense the condition of the tissues under her hands, becoming aware of the tensions, temperatures and sensitivities. The lighter effleurage strokes are used on the larger areas of the body, as well as to prepare and warm the tissues for stronger and deeper strokes. The deeper effleurage movements are usually used when the tissues are already somewhat familiar with the touch of the therapist.

The effect: Effleurage is relaxing and pain relieving, it improves blood and lymph circulation in the tissues, hence the effleurage strokes are the principle movements for easing fluid retention in tissues.

Effleurage movements at the end of the treatment are usually performed in very light strokes and finishing with a move down the spinal column. At the end of the massage these strokes are aimed to calm and please.

Contra-indication: Fluid retention that is caused by kidney or heart problems are not to be treated with massage.

Friction
Friction is performed by pressing the soft tissues with circular movements against the bones underneath. The fingers must not slide across the surface of the skin but the therapist's hand and the tissue under it move together so the real friction is to the tissues underneath the skin. The move can be as large as the tissue will allow. The pressure can be constant throughout the movement or it can change so that it becomes lighter or stronger during the movement. Once again, especially on the legs and limbs the pressure becomes stronger towards the middle of the movement and lightens at the end, and in the direction of venous circulation. Friction can be performed either with the whole hand or any part of the hand depending on the area treated. The thumbs will give a very strong deep stroke which can be used for strong muscle spasms. This movement can be performed with either one or both hands simultaneously. Fists can be used for very strong muscles, for example the gluteals. Friction is usually performed after effleurage. As a rule the tissues are first treated with large friction movement, and once the tissues soften and relax under the hands, deeper friction can be performed.

The effect: Friction stimulates circulation and tissue metabolism. It will relax the muscles, relieve pain, remove as well as prevent fibrosis forming in tissues.

With the friction movements one can also uphold or improve the elasticity of soft tissues.

Petrissage/Kneading

In the petrissage movement the muscle is lifted from its base, between the thumb and fingers or between the fingers and the base of the hand, and then squeeze across the muscle fibres. Petrissage movements follow venous circulation. This movement can be performed with both or one hand where the hand moves along the muscle or group of muscles, and the muscle should not return back to its base between movements. The very large and strong muscles, for example the quadriceps, are treated with the two-hand petrissage movement. The muscle is always lifted directly upwards from its bony base. The limitation of the movement is that flat muscles cannot be treated in this way; only long and narrow muscles can be lifted from their base.

The effect: Petrissage improves both the venous circulation and the lymph flow in the tissues, it improves the elasticity of the muscles and prevents possible fibrosis from developing.

Kneading, as a form of petrissage, is performed with smooth gliding, twisting movements over the skin – in rhythmical repetition with alternating hands.

The effect: These moves will relax the muscles, remove waste matter, and stimulate the blood and lymph flow.

Tapotement/Tappotage

Tapotement is performed with light, fast taps with fingers and wrists relaxed. It is called finger, fist, palm or fingertip tapotement depending on the part of the hand with which the tapping movement is performed. With tapotement it is important to be aware of the strength of the tapping, so that it does not cause pain or discomfort. Tapotement which is performed with the little finger side of the hand, with the wrists and elbows bent, is known as 'hacking'. It is powered by the movement of the lower arm. The fingers are relaxed and the tapotement is performed with both hands quickly alternating. 'Cupping' is performed with the fingers together, slightly bent so that the hand forms a cup. In this way an air cushion is created between the hand and the area to be treated and this softens the strength of the stroke. The wrist and the fingers are relaxed and the movements are made with alternating hands and used on larger areas of the body. With first tapotement or 'pounding' the hands are held lightly in a fist, with wrists relaxed. The movement is made with alternating fists, with the palm facing down. Fist tapotement is used on large thick muscles, for example the gluteus and the back of the thighs. Fingertip tapotement is performed with the tips of the fingers simultaneously or one fixed finger at a time. Fingertip tapotement or 'drumming' is usually used for facial and head massages. Tapotements are used relatively seldom in massage. Not to be used on areas of broken capillaries.

The effect: Tapotement movements expand surface capillaries, thus improving circulation in these areas. Cupping when performed on the back helps to relieve congestion and remove mucus from the respiratory area.

Vibration

Up and down vibrating movements are performed with the hand or fingers. For example vibration can be used on the back or shoulder muscles. Vibration movements penetrate deeply into the muscle tissues.

The effect: Vibration is mainly used for relaxing and relieving pain. Vibration movements are also used to clear mucus from the respiratory system.

* * * * * *

There are several methods of aromatherapy massage which have been developed by the various schools of aromatherapy. They are very often light stroking movements to stimulate the surface circulation in order to improve the absorption of the essential oils into the skin. These methods rely on the circulatory stimulation and the essential oils alone to perform the cleansing of waste matter from the body systems. Some aromatherapy treatments also include the use of pressure points as in acupressure to achieve the required result.

Sometimes these methods are not sufficient to clear congestion from muscles that have been in a tight spasm for long periods of time. For these types of problems and deeper tissue congestion more precise work on muscle tissue is necessary, which is used in the Ulla-Maija Grace aromatherapy massage sequence. For this, thorough knowledge of the muscular system and its functioning is very important.

* * * * * *

It is not possible to learn massage from books, and so I have not included the aromatherapy massage sequence in this book. The therapist needs to be on the receiving end of the treatment, during training to know what kind of touch or movement feels good and right, to be able to apply it in a treatment situation.

It is also important that the therapist learns to use her own body and energies correctly. This must be taught during the training period.

PHYSIOLOGICAL EFFECTS OF MASSAGE

These effects are difficult to assess individually, as so many areas are simultaneously influenced.

Physiological effects are achieved on the following levels:
* Mechanical through pressure and stretch.
* Chemical secretions through touch.
* Reflex reactions in the same way as in reflexology, but also via the dermatomes.

Psychological – relaxation will help to ease pain and relax muscle tensions.

Nervous – affecting the nervous system from the peripheral dermatome nerves to the Central Nervous System.

Skin
Mechanical
- opens sweat and sebaceous glands and may cause increase of these secretions.
- scarring can become softer as it is released from the underlying tissues.

Mechanical/Chemical
- even slight kneading causes the mechanical to become chemical, releasing histamines and serotonins which instigate vasodilation locally.

Reflex
- transmission of sensations into deeper tissues as in acupressure etc.
- dermatones/cuti-visceral influences.

Nerves
Mechanical/Psychological/Chemical
- calming the Central Nervous System (CNS) – messages are transmitted through the peripheral Nervous System (NS) and the effect is the relieving of pain, by releasing sedating chemicals.

The cuti-visceral effects via the dermatomes are transmitted from the peripheral nerves to the CNS and then to the visceral organs.

Reflex zones
Many of the effects of massage can be explained by these 'distance effects'.

Lungs
Tappotage and vibration is used to remove phlegm from the respiratory organs (emphysema etc.). This helps to assist and deepen respiration.

Blood
Studies have shown slight increases in the haemoglobin count about 1 hour after treatment.

Fatty tissues
No effect.

Bones/Skeleton
Bones and joints are indirectly affected by stimulating circulation to the bones thus aiding cell nourishment and metabolism, for example to an area of a fracture, though the massage is performed at a distance from the injury.

Circulation (Blood)
Improves local capillary / local venous / local arterial circulation. Increases the amount of blood pumped to the heart and causes slight changes in blood pressure.

Total arterial circulation is considered not to be affected by massage.

Venous circulation:
This can be speeded up towards the heart – but the pressure of massage strokes on other tissues on the other hand restricts it somewhat. The circulation in the massaged area increases for a while because the massage opens perhaps otherwise inactive capillaries in the area.

Arnot-Schultz rule

> "Mild stimulation will increase physiological activity and very strong activity will inhibit or totally stop activity."

Thus knowing the correct pressure in massage is of the utmost importance. With correct application it is possible to achieve a similar increase in circulation as occurs in exercise.

Massage releases vaso-activating substances which expand and open the capillaries.

Blood Pressure:
As massage expands the capillaries it temporarily causes *a reduction in the systolic and diastolic blood pressure* and a slight increase in the heart rate.

Metabolism

Production of urine is increased especially after abdominal massage.
Cellular metabolism is improved due to circulatory stimulation.

Visceral organs

Abdomen:

> Massage has a direct effect only on the intestines and the colon, any
> other effects on the viscera are due to reflex and dermatomes action.

Heart massage in **First Aid Only**.

Lymph

Circulation of lymph is dependent on external activity, e.g. gravity, muscle
contractions, passive moves or massage. If there are blockages in the deep
lymph ducts the lymph can move along the surface ducts. Studies show that
massage greatly increases the movement and circulation of lymph.

In paralysis, the lymph and tissue fluids collect, especially in the limbs.
Massage is considered to be more effective than physiotherapy and/or
electrical stimulation, for the removal of these types of congestion.

Lymphatic massage is a very specialist treatment *that requires long and
careful training*. In Europe and Scandinavia this specialist lymph treatment is
used to assist in lymphoedema after difficult operations, such as breast
cancer.

Muscle tissue

Massage has been found particularly beneficial to the muscle tissue. Trained
muscle recovers from effort faster if massaged.

Massage will cause the relaxation of muscle tension and spasms. Damaged
tissue e.g. separation of fibres, increased amount of fibrosis, enlarged blood
vessels and other pathological changes can be improved by massage in
experienced hands.

Massage has no effect on muscle atrophy, but the muscle can be kept 'fit'
and less stiff and with less fibre attachment and better circulation with
massage, in readiness for when and if nerve function is restored. In paralysis
the muscles become spastic, they contract very easily in reflex even from
slight irritation such as massage. Some forms of spastic muscles benefit from
massage.

Fibrosis is common in damaged, spastic and immobilized muscle. This causes contraction, reducing the mobility of muscles and joints. Massage can stretch the fibres and stop the formation of fibrosis and even break some fresh new fibroses.

Physiological pain

Pain studies on acupuncture and other therapies have revealed, according to the gate (control) theory, that the pain impulses, that travel in the thin, slow nerve fibres are stopped by creating sensations that travel in the larger and faster nerve fibres. Thus 'the gate' (in the CNS) is closed to the pain impulses. In massage this is achieved by the sensations created by the massage movements. Endorphins and encephalins are released during massage and are responsible for part of the pain relief in massage.

6 Client-Therapist Communication

Points to note before and during the first appointment:

* Discuss the reasons for seeking treatment while making the first appointment to eliminate illnesses that may be contra-indicated for aromatherapy (see contra-indications for massage and aromatherapy).
* Skin brushing is an excellent method of preparing the skin to absorb the essential oils during the treatment. It clears away any dead skin cells and also improves surface capillary circulation.
* Sometimes it may be advisable for the client to be on a short cleansing diet before starting a course of treatments to clear any congestion in the colon.
* For more severe constipation colon cleansing or irrigation may be the answer. This process can be assisted by herbal extracts or teas.

It is important that both the therapist and the client understand that the best results of treatment are gained through co-operation between the client and therapist. Only by 'looking each other in the eye' and being equal in working together can the health of the client be expected to improve. The therapist must accept that only the client knows where they hurt, that the client's understanding of their own needs must be respected, and the whole treatment is on the client's terms.

The use of a consultation sheet is of great importance. This should be explained to the client before filling in the form. It is a record of the initial communication that takes place between the client and the therapist. It also ensures that if anything should go wrong, the insurance company has written information of the client's condition at the beginning of the treatment. This is a safety precaution for both the therapist and client.

The record card covers information on the client's health (both past and present), medication etc., and is the basis on which the therapist decides which oils to choose for each treatment. Even now when the complementary therapies – including aromatherapy – are more widely known and accepted, the therapist still often gets clients who are at the verge of losing hope of any improvement in their condition or even of easing their pain. They have often been through all possible conventional treatments and come to another therapist as a last resort as they have 'nothing to lose'. The clients are often totally helpless and lacking the ability to help themselves. There may be anxiety and fear in possibly having to live with this pain for the rest of their lives. All of this sets great demands on the therapist's skill, tact and professionalism.

Having completed the consultation sheet and chosen the oils, the therapist will tell the client what to expect from the treatment – no promises of miracles, but a realistic aim/goal for the treatment should be made, and how many treatments may be necessary for the achievement of that goal.

The client should be told what to do before the treatment can start. (How much they need to undress, which way to get on the couch.) The therapist also needs to tell the client what to expect during the treatment; what the process of the treatment is.

The therapist should only be a *listener* to the many complaints that may come from the client regarding the previous treatments or carers and not join in the criticism. She should aim to bring the client out of negative past experiences and help towards a more positive approach to working together for the improvement of the condition.

It is important that the client has *confidence* in the abilities of the therapist. To some extent this can be achieved by the showing of appropriate diplomas and certificates of memberships in professional organisations. Naturally the training the therapist has is of great importance in her confidence and trust in her own knowledge and abilities as an aromatherapist. This confidence of course then shows in the approach and attitude towards the work and the clients.

Much importance needs to be placed on the training, and factual knowledge of the therapist, but an all important part of the work is also being a wise listener. We can hear with our ears the words that the client says but this is only some 10% of our communication. The therapist has to learn to listen to the needs of the client with her ears, eyes and heart. An empathetic approach will make the client feel comfortable and safe – not being judged or criticised. This empathy must not lead to sobbing with the client; a clear objective distance to the situation must be kept.

It is the therapist's role to assist the client in regaining their health, but at the same time she must remember that there is *no recipe for life. Each one of us is responsible for every word uttered and advice given. It is especially so in therapy*. There is a great tendency in the various fields of therapy even now to believe that one system is better than another, and strict rules of daily routine are given to the clients. This may give an already vulnerable client great feelings of failure and of having 'got it all wrong', not knowing or understanding anything and feeling guilty for their own illness.

I remember a client who wished to change her therapist. She could not be persuaded to discuss the matter with her therapist as she was too frightened to do so. She said she was afraid to go to her appointments for fear of the reprimands for not having been able to stick to her strict routine. She was also afraid to cancel as the therapist was so aggressive and domineering on the phone she did not have the courage to cancel the appointment. She had even tried not going to an appointment and was telephoned by the therapist and told in no uncertain terms what she was thought of, on top of which she was sent a bill.

In other words do not set the client impossible tasks. If they were able to stick to them, they probably would not need help. It is much more productive to guide the client gently into changing their habits – be it exercise, diet, sleep rhythm, overwork or whatever, and give them time to assimilate the changes.

One more point that will keep the client feeling confident in the abilities of the therapist is that the therapist knows her limitations. Thus the therapist knows when to refer the client for some other treatment if her own resources are not enough.

THE CLIENT

The client is the most important factor in this whole section as without her there would be no need for the treatment. The second most important factor is that the client and the therapist (and therapy) find each other acceptable. It is possible that communication between the two parties is not always supportive to the outcome of the treatment. If there is any dislike or unease from either party for whatever reason the treatment outcome is not going to be the best possible. It is therefore important that the client always finds a therapist that she is at ease with and can trust at all levels.

As an aromatherapy treatment of necessity starts with taking the case history, the client must be prepared to disclose this information. This will enable the therapist to choose the appropriate oils and to avoid those, if any, that are contra-indicated.

This initial talk will also cover the client's current situation and she may be asked questions on work, diet, exercise, etc. which are an integral part of

FACTORS AFFECTING THE OUTCOME OF TREATMENT

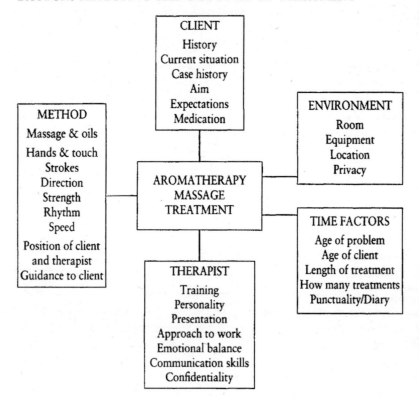

life and have an influence on health. This discussion will also tell the therapist the reason why the client has come to see her and help to set an appropriate aim for the treatment.

On each visit to the aromatherapist a record will be kept on the progress of the treatment. Sometimes the client will be given oils to use and other instructions to follow at home, and a record will also be kept of these. In this way at the end of the treatments one can enjoy the pleasant reading the progress often makes, as the goal is reached and many other surprising things may have happened.

THE THERAPIST

Education – the goal of the training is to give the necessary basic knowledge in anatomy, physiology, methodology, the essential and carrier oils, psychology, and of course the manual practices. No training can guarantee that a student will become a good therapist. The student requires many other traits, both internal and external which are necessary for a good, professional and successful therapist. A person working in health care requires certain psychological traits; she needs to have a fair amount of empathy, unselfishness, extroversion, but most of all she must possess the ability to work with and enjoy other people. She needs to be sensitive, but not so much so that the problems of the client become her own, as then the work becomes a burden and the therapy will suffer. The therapist must be able to, when necessary, encourage the client and help the client to trust herself and the treatment. The ability to listen is one of the most important skills, and an absolute necessity for the development of a good care situation. During the treatment, the therapist's time is only for the client. The therapist's own worries and pressures must not be apparent in the treatment situation. Having gained the trust of the client, *the therapist is bound by confidentiality*. NO information about the client, not even their name, must be taken outside the care situation. Therapy is a service profession, therefore, the client is always right. *The client is always the expert on their own situation*. The therapist needs to be polite and sensitive towards the client, punctual and precise in the treatment.

Appearance

We can transmit many messages with our appearance to those around us. White or pale clothing is an external sign of the health care profession. White clothes accentuate one of the most important aspects; cleanliness. In practice this means that the work clothes of the therapist have to be changed daily. The material must be easy to wash and iron and be made of natural fibres and of course, be loose enough so as not to hinder free movement.

During massage one works in very close proximity to the client. The work can cause the therapist to perspire, therefore she must be very aware of her own personal hygiene.

The most important tools of a massage therapist are her hands. They must always be washed immediately before and immediately after the treatment and if necessary also during the treatment. This constant washing dries the skin, so it is important to ensure that they are well moisturised. The skin of the hands must be healthy. *One must not give treatment if there is infection or cuts on the hands*. The nails must be short enough so that they cannot be felt on the client's skin. Watches, rings and other jewellery must be removed. Cold hands are unpleasant on the client's skin and must be warmed, for example during the wash with warm water.

MASSAGE AS A TREATMENT

Massage is always a dynamic process in which one needs to take into account many influences. These are the client, the therapist, the history and condition of the client and the environment. Massage can easily become a routine in which the same moves are repeated regardless of the client's needs. Successful treatment requires a goal and a plan. During massage the sensitive hands of the therapist can transmit many kinds of messages. There is also a need for verbal exchange of thoughts, emotions and experiences. For good results there is a need for continuous giving and receiving of information, co-operation and constant assessment and decision making. In this way each treatment becomes unique for each individual and the client's needs and wishes are the deciding factors in the massage.

Massage, just as any other treatment, aims at certain results. Before deciding on the goal the therapist must get to know the client's background and current condition. The background, one can find out from the client himself or notes sent by the doctor. Other important information is the client's age, occupation, previous illnesses and treatments. Certainly if the current illness, its symptoms, and the problems that it causes are visible, one can define the most obvious problem area and its severity, through observation and touch. The therapist must also take into account whether massage is a part of the client's wider treatment programme or whether it is the only treatment for her. From the gathered information the therapist then assesses the condition of the client and decides a plan and goal of the treatment. The goals of the treatment must be realistic. Progress is expressed in descriptions of the changes that occur in the client's condition from one treatment to the next. The therapist continuously reassesses the client's condition, the symptoms and changes in the original problems. In aromatherapy the aim of the treatment is to bring harmony to the body systems and feelings of the client.

As aromatherapy is such a complete treatment it is possible to have good results even with few treatments. How the client feels after each treatment is naturally dependent on the essential oils used, and the method used during the massage. The rhythm, the speed and the direction of the strokes should be adjusted to follow the overall effect of the essential oils for maximum benefit. The most important deciding factor on the style of the treatment is of course the wishes of the client. The slower, smoother and more continuous the strokes are the more relaxing and soothing the treatment. The more rapid the movements are the more stimulating the effect. Whatever the method and style of treatments there comes a time when the client will feel that a clear change is taking place.

This usually happens in weekly treatments around the 4th or 5th week. Up until then all has been fine. The client is feeling progressively better until that time. Then she may 'catch the flu' or have skin eruptions or some other adverse health reaction. This is what we call the Healing Crisis – the body has decided to start the cleansing from inside out, and it expresses itself in these ways. The best treatment then is to allow the body to do its work. It can be helped by clean light foods, plenty of fluids and essential oils in low doses as appropriate according to each person's needs.

TIME FACTORS

The treatment begins from the moment the client is greeted and welcomed. She should be made to feel comfortable and at ease immediately upon arrival. An important way of achieving this is by the therapist introducing herself to the client, by making it known how she wishes to be addressed and also how the client wished to be called. As the therapist always works with an appointment system there will be no waiting time, therefore the reserved time is totally devoted to the client.

Appointment records

The therapist must keep a clear diary of her appointments to ensure that the client is allocated sufficient time for the treatment. She should also give the client an appointment card or a clear indication in some other way of her allotted time.

It is a matter of mutual respect to stick to these times, and if either is late for an appointment, adjustment to the change of treatments must be made. In other words, if the therapist cannot keep to her timetable for any reason and the client's treatment is left short a reduction in the fee is appropriate. On the other hand if the client is late for her appointment a full fee will be charged for the reduced treatment.

The client can and should demand the therapist's total attention for the reserved time. The therapist needs to ensure that telephones and other possible interruptions are eliminated.

Such facts as the age of the client and how long they have had the problem, have a bearing on the length of each treatment and on how many treatments may be needed to achieve the set goal. Almost always with physical conditions the number of years the client has had the problem is directly connected to the number of treatments required. This rule does not appear to apply to problems in the emotional/psychological area as sometimes help can be found very rapidly for these.

CREATING A THERAPEUTIC ENVIRONMENT

In aromatherapy our aim is to really care for the client. They must feel like the most important person in the world for the duration of the treatment and their appointment. This makes some demands on the environment in which the treatment takes place.

It needs to be comfortable in many ways:

Comfort

Comfort means safety. The place must be easily accessible, even for clients with disabilities, and the equipment and furniture safe and appropriate. A comfortable atmosphere is created by using soft decoration that is easy on the eyes, gentle sounds that are soothing and lighting that is warm, but bright enough to see. The sheets and towels must be fresh and soft, and there need to be enough of them to keep the client covered and warm, as the client undressed may feel cold. The treatment room should also be warm, aired and airy.

Hygiene

There are also demands on the hygiene of the treatment place. Hygiene means that the room is thoroughly clean, not just dusted and the carpet vacuumed, but clean. The working surfaces, windows and carpets must be free of oil stains that so easily are an eyesore in aromatherapy treatment rooms. Each client has clean sheets or couch paper and clean towels. The dishes and equipment must be scrupulously clean and washed between clients, and each client is made a new fresh blend of oils (blends saved for the next client, or the same client for next time are never acceptable!). The therapist must wash her hands between each client twice – once before starting treatment and once after. (Sometimes it is necessary to wash one's hands during the treatment.) The therapist must be clean and wear clean, appropriate clothing and must keep her hands healthy and nails short.

Privacy

Privacy also sets demands on the place of treatment. This means that the client is not on view to outsiders and that there are no distracting noises and that you are not overheard. The telephone should not disturb the treatment. The confidentiality of the given information is guaranteed by keeping client records locked up. If the client wishes she can dress/undress alone or behind a screen and the parts that the client wishes to keep covered and untouched are respected.

Insurance

The therapist must display an up-to-date insurance certificate on the wall of the treatment room. All large professional aromatherapy organizations have them available for their member therapists.

FOLLOW-UP AND SUPPORTING TREATMENTS BY OTHER THERAPISTS AND AT HOME

The extent of the need to use the help of other therapists naturally depends on the severity and the type of problem treated in relationship to the type of training the therapist herself has received.

There is no current law that states the training requirements for any of the alternative and complementary therapies, excluding osteopathy, and the responsibility for the standards of the training is left to individual professional associations. It is up to the therapist to be properly trained and also to the client to check that the therapist is what they claim to be.

It is important to remember that giving advice in any area of health care is always a very delicate process of reading the client/patient's ability to accept advice and more to the point their ability to follow it. Very often the ability to follow disappears because of the severity of the instructions and how they are given. It is also possible that the slightest implication to an emotionally fragile client that they themselves may be responsible for the state they are in, will make them feel totally worthless and give up before they even get started.

Ann Coxon, neurologist, in her lecture at the IFA in 1990, very aptly said that "the strength of aromatherapy is in its nonverbal communication". Allowing the client to become familiar with their needs *from within themselves* ensures that any subsequent advice will be followed.

Every aromatherapist should be able to give guidance to the clients on the use of *essential oils at home* to support and continue the treatment between visits to the therapist.

Often advice is needed in the *dietary habits* of the client. We are all aware that nutrition is a key issue in our health and well being. *You cannot grow a healthy rose with soil that is poorly nourished. Similarly our bodies cannot create healthy cells to build a healthy body if the materials for the growth are of inferior quality.* If the therapist has no training in nutritional matters and there is need of more than common sense advice it is worth seeking help from a nutritionist.

Exercise is also of paramount importance for everyone, but in particular for those whose health is failing. This does not mean that everyone has to start hefty aerobic practices, quite the contrary. One of the very best exercises is a brisk walk in fresh air, long enough to give a feeling of warmth and enough exertion to make the heart beat a little faster than usual. Swimming and yoga are also excellent forms of exercise that are easily available to everyone without the need for an excessive amount of equipment or expense. These two are also good as there is no competition, and *each person proceeds and improves at their own pace according to their abilities.*

The most *important factor* in exercising, food and any method of improving health and wellbeing is that it is *regularly practised* for a long enough time. It takes a long time for the body to renew all its cells (it is said to take seven years) and each cell holds a memory of its old habits and has a tendency and wish to return to them. Perseverance in learning to form new habits is the only answer for continuous wellbeing and improvement of health.

Some aromatherapists have studied *counselling skills* and have the ability to practice this profession in its own right. It is a very skilled and delicate process and without the proper training must not be undertaken.

There are problems that an aromatherapist cannot successfully treat without the assistance of other experts. These include skeletal problems which need the hands of an *osteopath* or a *chiropractor. Homoeopathic* treatments are sometimes a faster route out of a problem, though there is controversy over the justification for the very high potencies sometimes used for treatments. A therapist should also be sufficiently aware of the signs that indicate a more serious problem that needs the attention of a *doctor.* For this the processes of how to communicate with the medical profession and the terminology used need to be correct and appropriate.

The Three 'R's

Rights – Respect – Responsibility
Man is a conscious being, one who has four levels of life existence:

The Physical Body
This represents the minerals of the world in plants and humans.

The Life Body

That which makes this whole world tick. Makes the seeds grow and know how to start, or birds to know when to fly south for the warmth or north to breed, or the sperm to fertilize the egg.

The Emotional Body

Or soul, where feelings and sensations are the rulers.

The Mind

The conscious thought processes that are the privilege of man only on this beautiful Earth of ours.

Man is first and foremost ruled by the laws of his nature. He cannot escape his physical and life body. He cannot avoid being influenced by the emotions and thought processes that are the products of his past experiences created within his life cycle.

What these experiences are depend on the society and the culture that he has lived in. Man lives as a member of these various cultures and societies and develops his personality to a great extent according to its teachings and laws. How he experiences himself and how conscious he is of his present state can and will influence his future. The more conscious man is of the fact that at all times he is free to choose the direction his life will take, the more he can and will influence all areas of his life.

One of the major areas that an aromatherapist, or any other therapist for that matter, can help a client in is in bringing the awareness that we are all capable, to a greater or lesser degree, of helping ourselves in so many ways. We do not need to be the victims of the past, or of old patterns of behaviour in health care, diet or any other area of life.

This freedom to choose one's path is also the foundation for being responsible for one's actions and life at all times. This could be called 'the eye of the needle that the camel has to pass through.' Each client and each therapist has rights and responsibilities to adhere to, including respect for each other.

Rights of the Client:

* To choose the type of treatment and therapist they feel is appropriate, and check the therapist's qualification.
* To tell only as much of the details of their history that they want to.
* To be the expert in the knowledge of their own bodies and when and where it hurts.

* To insist on the total attention of the therapist for the duration of the appointment.
* To discontinue the treatment any time they wish.
* To insist on the hygiene of the therapist, the room, the linen etc.

Rights of the Therapist:

* To choose the clients, according to the skills of the therapist and also likes/dislikes.
* To insist on a signature on a consultation sheet that states that the facts disclosed are true and accurate.
* That unless especially agreed or necessary the client comes alone to the treatment room.
* To discontinue the treatments when she feels appropriate.
* To insist on the client's hygiene: clean body, feet and clothes.

All rights lead to *Responsibilities*

Responsibilities of the Client:

* To check that the chosen therapist is properly trained
  * membership of organizations
  * insurance cover
  * diplomas and certificates should be on display
* To make sure that the therapist is given the facts she asks for that may be contradictory to the use of some oils or techniques. If they are not and something goes wrong the therapist's insurance will not cover it.
* In being the expert on one's own feelings and sensations also lies an opportunity and possibility to help oneself with the guidance of the therapist to improve the health of the body.
* To continue the treatments for improvement and to know that if the treatments are discontinued before the problem is fully resolved it may come back quite rapidly.

Responsibilities of the Therapist:

* To continually keep up with new knowledge and information on the professions – even after proper training is achieved. Though the best teacher in the practical side of the therapy is each client, it is still vital to keep up with all the new knowledge on the essential oils.

* To be properly insured and to use the consultation sheets correctly – both for the benefit of the client and the therapist.
* To be well enough versed in the basic guidance of nutrition, exercise and relaxation to be able to instruct the client, or to know other therapists or classes nearby that would be appropriate to the client.
* To know when to refer the client to some other treatment.

Respect:

In this three 'R' section the final 'R' stands for Respect, and the points made here apply both to the client and the therapist equally.

All of us, at all levels and walks of life, need to remember daily that each of us has the right to be respected as equal human beings. Our individuality, our consciousness is that which gives each of us a very special personal identity; that which enables us to make our imprint on the world. We need to respect everyone's right to their personal relationships (friendship, love) feelings and opinions. And most of all allow everyone to develop at their own pace according to their personal abilities and respect them for the effort that they put into each new day.

Does grace not mean the chance to start every day anew? Each step that we take towards being responsible for our health and well being, both physical and emotional, we can count as a new feather in our cap.

THERAPEUTIC TOUCH

The term therapeutic touch was first used by **Martha Rogers** and refers to a holistic form of care in which the client is helped to achieve a level of self understanding and confidence to activate and motivate her to help herself on the road to healing. The method used is a form of energy therapy in which the therapist intentionally assists the balancing of the client's energy field or aura, as it is described in the eastern traditions. Thus the client can find a way of adjusting her own life patterns and routines to make it whole again.

Rogers sees illness as important for development. Sometimes an illness is the only way in which an individual will become aware of her way of life and its effects.

In Rogers' theory man and environment are open energy fields which are in constant and simultaneous exchange of energy and expansion with the universe. Both are in a constant and irreversible process of change towards individualism and complexity.

There are many forms of hands-on therapy to which the term therapeutic touch could be applied. In theoretical terms and in nursing studies on the effect of touch, the difference between these methods lies in the intention or awareness of the therapists. In Rogers' theory of therapeutic touch the therapist consciously uses her hands to find imbalances in the energy field around the client which she then balances by moving energy from one area of the aura to another. She can also become a channel for the universal energy to boost a depleted energy field, or to remove excess energy.

The above description of therapeutic touch, in my opinion, assumes that the therapist is well versed in the energy flows within and without the human body. It also gives an impression that a therapist has a right to impose her will upon the client, to consciously change the energy flows. **Barbara Ann Brennan's** book 'Hands of Light' will give an idea of how much training is required for this.

* * * * * *

There are other approaches to therapeutic touch. In aromatherapy it is a hands-on-skin contact. This gentle stroking of the skin in itself is therapeutic, as touching one another has somehow become taboo. In this therapy situation you are allowed to receive touch and care without having to respond to it in any way.

Words of an old lady who had found aromatherapy, come to mind.

"I really am a very fortunate old lady as I have given myself permission to come to be cared for."

Therapeutic touch in this gentle massage treatment also refers to the touching of the skin all over and the effect it has on the nervous system. According to neurology this sends messages from the whole of the peripheral nervous system to the brain, which begins to secrete substances that are the body's own painkillers and hormones that make you feel good (endorphins and encephalins).

Therapeutic touch is also a matter of communication between the client and the therapist. This communication can be in non-verbal form and even without the physical touch. It can simply be a welcoming look or clear expression of approval that comes from the heart of the therapist. Love of another human being is the greatest of healers in all therapy situations.

Whatever the form that the therapeutic touch takes, the integrity of the therapist needs at all times to be under scrutiny. As a therapist it is very easy to begin to put one's own egoistic needs and goals before that which is best for the client. In our limited understanding of the universal realities it is not easy if at all possible to know what is best. So provided the therapist in her mind and heart aims and prays for the treatment to be for the best of the client as well as being a competent, fully trained therapist then she has fulfilled the requirements for therapeutic touch.

To be aware of the possible effects of touch and therapy challenges the therapist to be on her guard at all times, and to continuously develop as a therapist and as a human being.

7 Routes of Administration

SKIN

In aromatherapy the skin and its conditions is an important tool for the therapist in gaining information on the condition of the client and also a route of administration of the oils. These are absorbed into the body via the skin with the assistance of the sebum. The fat (lipid) soluble aromatic molecules dissolve into the sebum and pass through into the deeper layers of skin, where they are picked up by the blood and lymphatic systems and transported throughout the body.

Depending on the condition of the skin the absorption of the aromatic molecules into the deeper layers takes about 20 minutes. Rates of absorption are also dependent on the composition of oil. The lipid soluble short chain terpenes absorb fastest.

The ability for the skin to receive and absorb the oils can be influenced by improving the capillary circulation and removing of the dead keratinized layer of the surface. This can be achieved by cleaning the skin thoroughly (sauna if possible), dry brushing or peeling, exercise in fresh air or air baths in front of an open window.

Internal cleanliness is also vital to the responsiveness of the skin. The colon and intestines are the most important internal environments and naturally the food we eat will create that environment and affect its general condition. Growing a rosy glow on the skin needs as much care in nourishment as growing a beautiful rose.

The skin is a continuously renewing organ of the body. It acts as an interface between our internal and external environments and responds and reacts to changes in both. It has several functions:

It *protects* the body from external influences by its rapid rate of cell growth, thus helping to heal wounds and defend against poisons, ultraviolet rays, bacteria etc.

It *prevents* excessive loss of fluid from the body.

It also has a covering of non-pathogenic 'friendly' bacteria which *forms a protective barrier against invading pathogens* together with its acid-mantle of 7 pH.

It *regulates* the body temperature, keeping it warm by acting as an insulation (subcutaneous fat), raising of body heat to form a warm air cushion around the body (goose bumps), constricting of surface capillaries and cooling down by sweating.

It is a *sensory organ* for all kinds of touch, pain, hot, cold, caressing. For the therapist, the skin on her hands and fingers are the antennae, and eyes for detection of problem areas and other signs of the client/patient's condition. For the client the skin is an organ for receiving the sensations that the therapist's hands transmit.

The skin is responsible for approximately 2% of the total oxygen exchange.

In co-operation with the sun it creates vitamin D for the use of the body in the formation of bones.

The functioning of the sebaceous glands determine whether our skin is dry or moist – it protects from loss of fluid.

The skin and the nervous system are in direct contact with each other. In the foetus they are formed from the same epithelial tissue.

The condition of the skin will give the therapist some clues by which to help to decide on the oils to use for the treatment. To quote Shakespeare, the skin tells of not only the physiological conditions, but also of the mind.

'So changes the healthy skin of determination to the paleness of uncertainty.'

The skin reflects inner change, both physical and emotional. Colour is one indication of these changes. Here are some examples of how some colours reflect these:

Colour	Physical problem	Possible cause	Emotion
Bluish	Heart/circulation	Disease, smoking	Cold
Pale/white	Arthritis Anaemia	Steroids	Shock, fear, rage
Yellow/brown	Kidney infection Jaundice		
Reddish	Couperose High blood pressure	Liver Hereditary, diet	Anger Embarrassment

Colour	Physical problem	Possible cause	Emotion
Yellow/green	Sickness Gall/bile	Bacteria	Bitter/sour
Grey	Poor breathing	Smoking Lack of exercise	Depression Negativity
	Asthma Kidneys	Dysfunction	

Skin texture

Texture	Physical problem	Possible cause
Sandpapery	Stagnation	Poor elimination
Fluidy/bloated	Lack of sensation	Hormonal imbalance Nervous system dysfunction
Dry/does not perspire	Blocked sweat glands	Holding on to emotions
Blocked non-functioning due to physiological or emotional problems	Needs lungs strengthened, Breath deepened	
Acne	Hormonal imbalance Intestine candida/ elimination Lungs/asthma	Stress Strong antibiotic medication Poor diet Poor respiration

Skin Temperature

Temperature	Possible cause
Hot	High blood pressure Infection Cancer/localised heat Excessive activity
Cold	Lack of activity Circulation Thyroid/hypothyroid condition

Other influences

Influence	Effects
Hormones	Boils, spots, patches
Heat	Drying, wrinkles, heat rash
Moisture	Favourable/soft, smooth skin
Smoke/pollution	Ageing, greying, wrinkles
Alcohol	Redness, bloatedness (kidneys), couperose
Strong medication	Poor elimination, weakened function, pores blocked from dead cells
Stress	Dry, tight
Air conditioning	Dry, tight

When the body is balanced problems disappear.

The above are meant as a guide only and are by no means conclusive. Once again each client is an individual and there are no hard and fast rules. A therapist needs to be a detective and learn to read the obvious physical signs and the more subtle suggestions, and put them all together to reach the correct conclusion.

To improve the absorbtion of the essential oils through the skin daily dry brushing is recommended and also steam baths or saunas to clear blocked pores. Exercise and deep breathing will also help to improve the condition of the skin.

THE RESPIRATORY SYSTEM

The Upper Respiratory Tract

THE NOSE is the organ of olfaction and respiration. The nose cleanses, warms and moistens the inhaled air. Coarsest impurities get caught in the cilia and smaller, in the mucus.

Mucus runs from the nasal cavities and the bronchi into the throat and gets swallowed. The warming is done by the dense capillary network in the mucous membrane. The tear ducts that bring tears from the eye connect with the inferior concha nasalis. The ear duct connects with the nasopharynx.

THE PHARYNX situated behind the nose, is divided into three parts and contains the adenoids and tonsils as a first lymphoid defence system in the respiratory tract.

113

THE LARYNX or the voice box is situated between the pharynx and the trachea. It is instrumental in producing sound and contains the epiglottis which prevents food from entering the trachea during swallowing.

THE TRACHEA or the wind pipe continues from the larynx and divides into two to become the *lower respiratory tract*.

The Lower Respiratory Tract

THE RIGHT AND LEFT BRONCHI which enter the lungs are formed by the bronchial tubes, which pass through the *hilus pulmonis* into the lungs where they divide again and become bronchioles.

THE BRONCHIOLES end in 10 segments in each lung. They further divide, and the smallest bronchioles end in alveoli, the very last extremities of the lungs, which are in direct contact with the capillaries.

THE LUNGS are situated in the thoracic cavity which is made up of the ribcage and the diaphragm. These are responsible for the creation of the movement which facilitates the respiratory cycle. Ventilation is the exchange of the air between the external environment and the respiratory system. This process is assisted by the musculature of the diaphragm, throat, chest and abdomen. In external respiration, the gaseous exchange takes place at the alveolar/ capillary level of the lungs. During this carbon dioxide is removed from the blood to the lungs and new oxygen is brought into the blood from the lungs. The gaseous exchange of the alveolar air and blood is based on the fact that gases always move from greater to smaller pressure.

The oxygen brought by the ventilation, external respiration into the alveoli and then into the capillaries, is carried around the body connected to the iron atoms in the haemoglobin.

The external respiration becomes internal or cellular respiration at the cellular level, where arterial blood brings fresh oxygen to the cells and removes carbon dioxide as waste from the cells.

The breathing control centre is located in the *medulla oblongata*, but ventilation is also influenced by many other factors, e.g. the chemical composition of the blood (whether it contains enough oxygen). Perhaps we could speculate that *Boswellia carterii* deepens the breathing by influencing the control centre via the blood. Ventilation is also affected by neuro-impulses from the cortex, the muscles and the skin. Does the deepening breath during massage occur as a direct result of the stimulation of the sensory receptors on the skin?

The respiratory system plays a very important role in aromatherapy. The fine volatile airborne molecules of the essential oils get carried into the lungs with the inspired air, and with the external and internal respiration, particles of it get absorbed into the bloodstream. Depending on the structure of the essential oil it begins to work on any invading bacterium or virus in the respiratory tract itself. We know that the terpenes are the least water soluble particles of the essential oils and the further the oxidation process goes the more water soluble they become (with the exception of the esters). Therefore we can assume that the alcohols, aldehydes, acids, ketones, lactones and coumarins are more readily absorbed through respiration than the terpenes.

There is an interesting recent study by **Professor G. Buchbauer** of the pharmacology department of the University of Vienna, on the effect of inhaled cineole oxide as a circulatory stimulant of the brain. He compared the results of inhalation of cineole for 20 minutes by a group of people with a normal sense of smell, to that of a group of people with no sense of smell. The behaviour of both groups changed in the same way. The results showed that with the first group the greatest increase in the blood circulation was in the side and upper sections of the cortex, and not so strongly elsewhere on the cortex. The stimulation of the areas of the cortex for the second group was in the side and the frontal lobes.

Whether the results of this test show that the effect is through respiration or olfaction is not clear. Professor Buchbauer maintains that aromatherapy is only acceptable as a therapy form via inhalation.

We know that the aromatic molecules carry potential information to affect emotions and moods via olfaction. We also know that the mucous membrane in the respiratory tract helps the absorption of the essential oils into the bloodstream, and also that the mucus is secreted continuously and swallowed into the digestive tract. Without further information we can only speculate on the route by which the stimulation of the cortex has occurred.

It would seem feasible that the more water soluble molecules would be more easily absorbed into the fluidy membranes of the respiratory tract and the less water soluble particles such as the terpenes in *Pinus sylvestris* and *Citrus limon* would work directly as antiseptics of the air in the tract.

THE OLFACTORY SYSTEM

The olfactory system is very sensitive and complex, with structures which integrate and create a double mechanism of response/reaction at the psychological and physiological levels.

Humans have various levels of osmia (the perception of odour). NORMOSMIC people have a so called normal level of perception of fragrance.

OLIGOSMIC people have a decreased level of fragrance perception and have more difficulty in detecting smells.

ANOSMIC people have no perception of fragrance. This may be due to congenital factors, or the mucous membrane may have been destroyed by strong chemical substances or manual intervention by operations. Temporary loss of osmia could be due to inflamed or blocked sinuses. Specific anosmia to certain substances is also a common occurrence.

CACOSMIC people perceive pleasant odours as unpleasant; this can be the result of psychological illness or disturbance.

The *quantitative* detection of each and every odour molecule is innate, depending on the sensitivity of the individual and does not change during life, nor is there any correlation between similar molecules, whereas the *qualitative* appreciation of odours is acquired during life through attraction or repulsion. Each of us has our own personal reference chart of odours and perception. The detection of various odour molecules vary from person to person. As the receptor cells in the olfactory mucous membrane are regenerative, the sense of smell can be trained as the cells renew themselves. Preference to different smells varies between various ethnic groups within a country and also between peoples in different parts of the world.

The olfactory system begins as part of the respiratory system in the nose, where the olfactory mucous membrane is situated at the top of the nasal cavity. The mucous membrane covers an area of two or three square cm. It contains the olfactory receptor cells, each of which have several receptors, making the total number of receptors around three hundred billion!

The aromatic molecules enter the nose with the inhaled air and are absorbed into the mucous membrane. This part of the process of smelling is aptly called "*captivation*". Here each molecule occupies a specific receptor site and emits the potential information, a message, which is then transmitted as electrical excitation along the olfactory neurons.

These messages go through various processes; *amplification* of the raw information at the level of the olfactory bulb, *refining* the message and *discrimination* for quantity of fragrance and quality of the types of molecules, *modification* of the message and finally *integration* of the message creating a *subconscious sensation* and *conscious picture* in the cortex. If the odour is familiar, e.g. lemon, a conscious picture of the fruit is formed by the original potential information carried by the molecules.

The integration of the message seems specifically to be in the above order. This can be demonstrated by the following:

If in a dramatic situation, e.g. an accident, there is an unknown aroma in the air, in the future that same aroma will always first bring into consciousness the sensations and feelings at the scene of the original situation. Even after the source of the odorous substance later becomes known and recognized (e.g. lemon scent – lemon fruit), the subconscious sensations and feelings always precede the conscious picture the source of the smell forms in the mind.

There are several properties of the aromatic molecules that help in the discrimination of the odours. These include:

- the electrical characteristics of the compounds, that is whether they are electron donors or electron acceptors in air or whether they are hydroxyl compounds and disassociate in water;
- the spatial structure of the molecule. This is the three dimensional shape the molecule occupies in space – an isomer (mirror image) of a molecule will give information of a different odour to the olfactory sense;
- polar and apolar (water solubility) structure affects the speed in which the molecules get absorbed into the fluidy mucous membrane and therefore the speed of their detection and recognition;
- the molecular weight (the number of protons and neutrons in the nucleus of each atom) has an effect on the discrimination. The smaller the molecular weight, the more easily it is absorbed.

The sense of smell 'tires' easily. If the amount of odour is too great the receptors become saturated and recognition of the different aromas becomes difficult. If too much of one type of aroma, e.g. in perfume is used, the particular receptors that recognize those aromatic molecules become saturated and the smell can no longer be detected. We all know the phenomenon of the fine lady with the overpowering perfume who can no longer smell herself and keeps adding more of it, while those around her are suffocating.

Physical and Psychological Reactions

Different smells cause different reactions. Using the example of the lemon again, the fresh smell of lemons may cause you to start to salivate. Our sense of smell can also be a warning to us. Just think of food (e.g. an egg) that has gone bad – as soon as you break the shell, even before your consciousness says 'its bad' your stomach reacts by retching and wanting to vomit.

The sense of smell is the only sense in which the information to the CNS does not travel via the thalamus. The olfactory tract from the olfactory bulb ends on the medical surface of the temporal lobe, which contains the primary olfactory area, which is directly connected with the limbic area. The CNS parts that control the autonomic NS functions cannot anatomically be separated from the other parts of the CNS. Stimulating the hypothalamus and the limbic area will affect such intangible aspects as memory, emotion, and psyche, as well as having physical effects on the endocrine and autonomic nervous systems, which basically dictate the day-to-day functioning of our body; heart rate, body temperature, hunger, thirst and hormone production.

The psychological reactions that smelling an odour create are always at two stages.

1. Immediate – the feeling of attraction or repulsion to the smell.
2. Delayed – psychological reactions of changing moods or attitudes.

The *effects* of treating via the olfaction can be seen as *objective* in the change of cardiac or respiratory rhythm and modification of brain wave patterns, and *subjective* in the feeling of wellbeing and changes in behavioural patterns.

Physical problems can be treated indirectly via olfaction. This works by affecting the various body systems by influencing the CNS with odours, increasing the general feeling of wellbeing and influencing the working of the endocrine glands, nervous system and the cardiac and circulatory systems.

8 Conditions

This section of the book looks at the various problems that an aromatherapist could be asked to treat. The list is by no means complete, but is based on my own experience of ten years as a therapist and six years as a teacher of professional aromatherapy. During this time my own case histories cover close to ten thousand treatments, and treatments in the case studies that the students have produced for me to read amount to over five thousand.

At all times we must remember the individual needs of each of the clients and therefore it is difficult to give recipes for the problems. In some cases there are guides to which essential oils to use and in some cases where the physical problem needs very specific oils, exact recipes are included.

PAIN

Human pain can be due to many different causes and take a multitude forms. Each individual experiences pain in her own unique way. Pain that is a mere twinge to some may be absolute agony to others. Looking at pain in depth would fill a whole book, so here we only touch the surface of this subject.

The reasons for pain are usually grouped into four areas: physical, emotional, social and spiritual (Twycross and Lack 1983).

Physical pain is caused by injury, illness or a physical reaction to an emotional or spiritual hurt or social rules.

Emotional/Psychological pain may be grief, sorrow, embarrassment, indignation, depression, anxiety or psychological illness.

Social/Cultural pain: usually this type of pain is caused by actions or rituals that introduce each member of society to a physical or emotional pain as a part of their role in that society. It can also be pain due to social pressures in multi-cultural areas or pain due to an accepted form of punishment in a society.

Spiritual pain is caused by severe religious rules that build feelings of guilt, inferiority and fear of dying, or punishment by God.

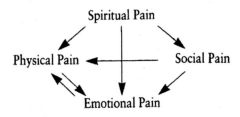

In Aromatherapy we can directly relieve the physical and emotional pain.

Physical pain can be relieved both by massage and essential oils. Gentle massage strokes can inhibit the pain/sensations by closing the 'gate' ('the Gate Control' theory) and stopping the pain impulses being transmitted to the cerebral cortex. The areas massaged or stroked need not be the affected parts and so even those who cannot have full massages can benefit from this gentle form of treatment.

Massage can also relieve pain *in situ* if the pain is caused by muscle spasm. Muscle can only contract in one way irrespective of whether the contraction is caused by physical effort (e.g. exercise) or emotional reasons (e.g. pulling shoulders up to ears in fear). Using deeper and stronger strokes it is possible to release muscle fibres that are 'glued' together with lactic acid. Massage can also release pain in stiff joints by bringing back elasticity to the muscles moving them and thus allowing freer movement of the joints.

The essential oils relieve pain in several ways. Some oils are analgesic in action and are often applied locally to the painful area e.g. *Mentha piperita* (peppermint) for sciatica or *Eugenia caryophyllus* (clove) for toothache. It can almost be said that each of the oils has some pain-relieving action depending on its application;

Anti-inflammatory oils work by removing the cause of the pain, the inflammation.

Rheumatic pain	–	*Origanum majorana* (marjoram)
Rheumatic inflammation/ painful joints	–	*Helichrysum italicum* (Italian everlasting)

Antispasmodic oils are directed to the area of the spasm, and chosen for each type of different spasms.

Muscular	–	*Lavandula angustifolia* (lavender)
		• high esters
		Pelargonium × asperum (geranium)
Menstrual	–	*Salvia sclarea* (clary sage)
		Ocimum basilicum var. basilicum (basil)
		Artemisia dracunculus (tarragon)

The reasons for emotional pain are not always clear even to the one feeling the pain, or it is too difficult to express. Often we need to choose the oils for this purpose on a general basis:

Grief/sorrow	–	*Rosa damascena* (rose)
		Origanum majorana (marjoram)
Anxiety/panic	–	*Cananga odorata* (ylang ylang)
		Melissa officinalis (melissa)
Fear	–	*Chamaemelum nobile* (Roman chamomile)
		Lavandula angustifolia (lavender)
Inferiority	–	*Jasminum officinale* (jasmine)
		Santalum album (sandalwood)

When treating people in much emotional pain, rose is always a useful choice, but in a very low dilution. One drop of steam-distilled *Rosa damascena* in 30–50 ml carrier oil is quite sufficient. The low dilution rule applies to all emotional pain. The oils are always clearly more effective in these areas when used in small quantities.

CONDITIONS OF THE RESPIRATORY SYSTEM

A brief look at this system was made in chapter 7. The most common problems in this area are easy to treat with aromatherapy in the form of inhalations and rubs. At times of cold and 'flu' epidemics the essential oils of *Pinus sylvestris* (pine), *Eucalyptus radiata* (Australian eucalyptus) and *Eucalyptus globulus*, *Thymus vulgaris* (thyme), *Citrus limon* (lemon) and

Citrus paradisi (grapefruit) keep room air clean of bacteria and reduce the spread of infection.

The Common Cold

The name common cold is given to a number of symptoms created by over a hundred different viruses. No 'cure' has been found for these. It seems that one should not even try to find such a cure as the symptoms are a sign that the body is responding to and learning from the invading virus. Once it has learned to 'cope' with the invader it knows how to handle it the next time it attacks.

We can ease the discomfort of a cold and sometimes help the body to be clear of it sooner by using the essential oils. Relieve nasal congestion and fight bacteria by using *Mentha piperita* (peppermint) and *Thymus vulgaris ct. linalol* or *Thujanol* (thyme) in an inhalation:

* two drops of each in a bowl of hot water repeated 3–4 times a day.

Other oils for this purpose could be *Rosmarinus pyramidalis* (rosemary), *Pinus sylvestris* (pine), *Picea mariana* (black spruce) and *Citrus limon* (lemon).

In addition to the inhalations it is good to use *Melaleuca alternifolia* (tea-tree), *Eucalyptus radiata* (Australian eucalyptus) or *Boswellia carterii* (Frankincense) in a 2–3% rub on the chest for continued inhalation (the heat of the body will help the vapour to rise from the skin) of these anti-bacterial oils. They also improve the body's own defences by stimulating the immune system.

Influenza or 'flu' is a viral infection by a specific virus. Its symptoms are more severe and often include fever and aching muscles and joints. The above treatments apply, but more emphasis is needed on the *Melaleuca alternifolia* (tea-tree) and other immunostimulant oils.

Fever is a sign of the body doing what it should, and as long as the temperature does not become dangerously high or continue for more than 48 hours it should be left to run its course. *Mentha piperita* (peppermint) will help to reduce the fever (not for young children and babies) and at the same time ease congestion.

Muscular and joint paints can be relieved by warming rubs or baths with *Origanum majorana* (marjoram), with *Citrus limon* (lemon) to assist the elimination of waste from the body and also to cheer the mind in the misery of the situation.

Pharyngitis and Laryngitis

These can also be helped with inhalations or rubs, prepared as above, on the lymph glands on the neck, or by using the oils as a gargle;

* Dilute 2 drops of *Thymus vulgaris ct l.* or *thuj.* (thyme) and 2 drops of *Melaleuca alternifolia* (tea-tree) in a small amount of alcohol (e.g. 5ml vodka), mix half of it into a glass of warm water and gargle. Repeat 2–3 times a day.

Tonsilitis and Adenoiditis

These will respond to *Eucalyptus radiata* (Australian eucalyptus) and *Laurus nobilis* (bay leaf) either cutaneously or as a gargle.

Bronchitis

Treatment of bronchitis needs an oil that will help to bring up the mucus created by the increased secretions due to the bacterial infection, smoking or air pollution. The best oils for this are the already mentioned eucalyptuses, *Cupressus sempervirens* (cypress), *Thymus vulgaris* (thyme) as above and *Origanum majorana* (marjoram).

* The oils need to be diluted to 5% and applied 3–5 times a day on the chest and back as well as using them in an inhalation.

* * * * * *

There are some other common conditions of the respiratory tract that an aromatherapist is often asked to ease.

Hay fever

Successful and lasting treatment of hay fever is a long process. It needs the immediate relief from symptoms that can be found from homoeopathic remedies, and the body's own healthy defence system needs building up by a careful dietary plan, which can be assisted with the immunostimulant essential oils already mentioned earlier in this chapter.

Sinusitis

This is best treated with inhalations of *Mentha piperita* (peppermint) and *Thymus vulgaris* (thyme), *Eucalyptus radiata* (Australian eucalyptus) or *Eucalyptus globulus* to reduce the inflammation of the mucous membranes and

123

to fight off the invading bacteria. It is also helpful to use the pressure points on and around the cheekbones to help drain the sinuses.

Asthma

First a caution on treating asthma sufferers. Test the oil to be used by inhaling the oil quickly to see if it causes a reaction. The most successful oil for asthma treatment has been *Ravensara* in massage and as a rub. Inhaling the ravensara straight from the bottle or putting one drop on the sternum will rapidly bring relief from the feeling of tightness and discomfort.

Other oils that can also bring relief to the symptoms of the above problems:

*   For the very young or frail *Lavandula angustifolia* (lavender) and *Aniba rosaeodora* (rosewood).

*   The above two and *Citrus aurantium ssp. aurantium neroli* (orange flower) for the asthma sufferers to relieve the stress and anxiety that so often is a companion in these problems.

* * * * * *

Unless the aromatherapist has medical or doctor's training, the more severe respiratory tract problems need to be left for the medical profession to treat, and providing they agree, the above oils can be used to ease the conditions in support of the more conventional treatments.

THE DIGESTIVE SYSTEM

In the digestive tract the food ingested is transformed into a suitable composition to be absorbed into the body organisms. The digestive tract begins in the mouth and continues as a mucus lined 'tube' through the body, changing its form and function as necessary along the way. It is a processing plant for the intake of nourishment and disposal of waste.

Digestion of food in the tract is assisted initially in the mouth by chewing and saliva, then in the stomach by the churning muscle action and the gastric juices secreted by the gastric glands. The environment of the stomach is acid pH 1–2.5. From the stomach the semi-digested food moves into the very alkaline duodenum, pH 7–8. It is in the beginning of the duodenum where the duodenal or peptic ulcers occur. This is said to be due to the malfunction of the mucus and acid secreting cells in the stomach. Often the occurrence of the duodenal ulcers is also related to high stress levels. The walls of the duodenum and ileum secrete digestive enzymes which help to break down the foods to enable absorption and completing the digestive process.

The small intestine follows next in the digestive tract. The lining surface is covered by villi (projections). The villi contain a network of lymphatic and blood vessels which absorb the, by now, highly 'processed' foods into the body. Food material that is not digested in the small intestine is 'pushed' by the peristaltic action into the large intestine. Protruding at the beginning of the large intestine is the appendix which contains lymphoid tissue. Some nutrients are still absorbed from the large intestine, but mainly water is absorbed to solidify the faeces. There is also some microbial activity in the large intestine in synthesizing folic acid and vitamin K, and fermentation of the unabsorbed nutrients.

Passing the food residues out of the intestine is initiated by new food in the stomach. It causes a contraction in the transverse colon that pushes food forward into the descending colon and so the material already there is pushed on. Repeated voluntary retention of faeces can cause constipation.

The functions of the digestive tract is assisted by the accessory organs. Illnesses of the accessory organs, the liver, the pancreas, and the gall bladder, are not in the scope of the aromatherapist to treat alone, but need the guidance of a doctor.

On the other hand, if there is only a slight sluggishness in the organs they can be stimulated to function better, using the appropriate oils.

CONDITIONS OF THE DIGESTIVE SYSTEM

Candida albicans

The colonisation of candida albicans in the intestines is nowadays a very common problem with people of all ages. This is believed to be greatly due to the excessive use of antibiotics which destroy the friendly intestinal bacteria together with the invading ones. If the problem becomes very severe the absorption of nutrients is reduced. This can lead to allergies or food sensitivities, bloatedness etc. The candida can also spread in the bloodstream throughout the body and invade other mucous membranes, bringing with it a multitude of problems.

When the candida is severe it is difficult to treat without the assistance of an experienced therapist, and even then it needs great willpower and perseverance to succeed and successfully keep the problem from recurring.

* The basis of the treatment is literally to starve the candida to death by removing all carbohydrates from the diet. The candida thrives on all kinds of sugar and yeast products so anything containing any kind of sugar is an ABSOLUTE NO!

I have experienced a very severe spread of candida and after three months of total abstinence of any sugars, a teaspoon of lemon juice in a glass of water tasted like sugar water. We are not aware of how much hidden sugar there is in our daily diet.

* The most important essential oil to assist in the treatment of candida is *Melaleuca alternifolia* (tea-tree), which contains at least 25% of terpinene-4-ol alcohol. This will destroy the candida yeast and improve the body's own defence mechanism. It can be used rectally as a pessary or applied cutaneously.

* A very uncomfortable symptom of this invasion in women is vaginal thrush. This can be treated very successfully with washes and a blend of essential oils.

For the wash dissolve 3 heaped tablespoons of pure sea salt in 2–3 litres of as hot water as the sensitive skin in the genital area will tolerate, and wash well the external areas and as deep into the vagina as you can. Then apply the following blend to the entire area:

	2 drops *Melaleuca alternifolia* (tea-tree)
	2 drops *Aniba rosaeodora* (rosewood)
or	2 drops *Thymus vulgaris ct linalol* (thyme)
	2 drops *Matricaria recutita* (German chamomile)
	2 drops *Picea mariana* (black spruce)
	10 ml of carrier oil

If itching is very severe one drop of *Mentha piperita* can be added to the blend.

Washing and the application of the oil should be repeated as often as the irritation occurs. The whole of the blend can be used up in one day, and if the problem persists the next day repeat the process. So far I do not know of cases in which it has lasted longer than two to three days if this routine is strictly followed.

Candida albicans can also be found in the mouth. Good treatment for this is to make a mouth gargle with some or all of the above essential oils. First blend the essential oils in 10 ml of vodka and mix well and add 40 mls of water. Use 20 drops in a glass of water for a gargle several times a day. Eating raw garlic will also help to clear the fungus.

Crohns disease
Some students both in England and in Finland have reported excellent results in relieving the discomfort of this disease using *Cananga odorata* and *Lavandula angustifolia*.

Coeliac disease
Coeliac disease is an allergy to gluten in grains. It leads to inhibition of the absorbtion of nutrients in the small intestine. The natural treatment for this is to leave the gluten out of the diet and strengthen the immunity and body's defences back to normal levels.

Cold sores
Treat Herpes simplex or cold sores and ulcers in the mouth by putting one drop of *Ravensara aromatica* or *Melaleuca alternifolia* (tea-tree) neat on the sore 3–4 times a day.

Constipation
Constipation can be caused by habitual delaying of evacuating the faeces, by low roughage foods and lack of exercise. It can also be a sign of emotional "holding". Whatever the cause the result is the same, the colon gets blocked and congested and when finally the evacuation is attempted it does not occur or can be very painful and cause haemorrhoids. Much attention to diet is needed in these cases. A very good first aid to constipation is the use of crushed linseed seeds as a dietary supplement. This is particularly good as it will increase the roughage in the colon and build up the mucous membrane in the colon, thus helping the evacuation. Regular exercise, like walking, regular meal times and unhurried, well chewed meals are also a necessity for the proper functioning of the colon.

The best essential oil for constipation is *Ocimum basilicum var. basilicum* 3% dilution massaged on the colon reflex on the soles of the feet, lower back and abdomen 2–3 times a day up to ten days if necessary.

Diabetes

Diabetes patients can be treated with aromatherapy safely providing cautions are heeded. If the patient is using insulin, essential oils that effect the pancreatic function should be avoided.

I have received no reports from my own clients or from any students of adverse reactions to aromatherapy treatment. The clients themselves make sure they check their blood sugar levels after treatments, and no fluctuations have been recorded due to the treatments.

Clients who are on dietary control can benefit from all of the essential oils and in particular those that improve the liver and pancreatic functions.

Gastric problems

Gastric problems in the stomach and the duodenum, commonly named gastritis, can be eased by using the essential oils of *Citrus aurantium petitgrain* (petitgrain) as below for heartburn.

Haemorrhoids

Haemorrhoids are related to constipation. The discomfort and pain that they cause can be relieved by daily use of the following essential oil blend.

> 20 drops *Cupressus sempervirens* (cypress)
> 20 drops *Melaleuca quinquinervia* (niaouli)
> 20 *Citrus limon* (lemon)
> 50 ml carrier gel or oil

Blend to be used locally two/three times a day for 3–7 days and then when required.

As alternatives for the above oils you can use *Pogostemon cablin* (patchouli) and *Eucalyptus citriodora* (citrus scented eucalyptus).

Pessaries in the same proportion with the above oils can be made in cocoa butter and used rectally, 2–3 pessaries daily.

Halitosis

Halitosis or bad breath can occur even if teeth are perfectly healthy. The problem is lower in the digestive tract, mostly in the intestine. It can be caused by difficulties of absorbtion from the small intestine due to coeliac disease or candidal infection or it could be due to constipation. Each one of these needs to be treated according to the form the problem takes.

Heartburn and indigestion

Heartburn and indigestion are common problems and can be eased by applying 3–5% dilution of *Mentha piperita*, *Citrus limon* (lemon) or *Citrus reticulata* (mandarin) locally to the solar plexus area two or three times a day until better.

Hiatus hernia

Hiatus hernia cannot be treated as such with aromatherapy but sufferers of this condition find relief of the symptoms when treated with aromatherapy. The oils for each case are chosen on the basis of the other needs of the client. If the client finds it difficult to lie on the abdomen the situation can be eased by using pillows to support the body.

Irritable Bowel Syndrome

Irritable Bowel Syndrome is a condition in which the bowel movement is intermittently constipated or like diarrhoea. No cause has been found for this but it is clearly related to stress and anxiety and triggered by some foods e.g. white flour. The condition is eased by treating the anxiety and stress with oils suitable for the client/temperament and recognizing and eliminating the offending foods.

Nausea

Nausea and travel sickness can be eased by inhaling *Mentha piperita* or applying it or *Citrus reticulata* (mandarin) on the solar plexus. Ginger drinks or biscuits are also good for easing nausea.

* * * * * *

All serious conditions of the digestive tract or the accessory organs need the attention of a doctor.

SKIN

The human face is a book of life. It tells of health, joys and sorrows.

> "True beauty is a ray, that is born of the most holy spirit and alights the body in the same way as life arises from the depths of the earth and gives colour and aroma to the flower."
>
> Kahlil Gibran 'Broken Wings'

Skin is a dynamic organ. The epidermis, the outer layer, is the result of the work of the deeper base layer where the plump new cells are born. The best way to keep a healthy glowing skin is to make sure that the body is well nourished and has sufficient building materials for healthy new cells.

This as we know is not always possible, and in our current living environments it is not even enough. We need to pay attention to the skin from the outside also. The skin is a veritable garden of various living organisms and on a healthy skin these are friendly and do not cause problems. The 'friendly' bacteria prefer an acid condition. In aromatherapy the use of carrier oils that contain large quantities of essential fatty acids will assist the skin care a great deal, provided good quality, fresh oils are used. Especially good for damaged skin are *Rosa rubiginosa*, *Evening Primrose* and *Jojoba*.

The essential oils work on the skin in many ways and on many levels.

* They improve the cellular regeneration and make the skin more dynamic by improving the metabolism. Oils effective in this are *Citrus aurantium* flowers (neroli), *Lavandula angustifolia* (lavender), and *Melaleuca alternifolia* (tea-tree).

* The essential oils aid the lymphatic function both in the ducts and the nodes, thus preventing the build up of waste matter by improving its elimination: *Cupressus sempervirens* (cypress) and *Pelargonium × asperum* (geranium).

* Some essential oils improve the capillary circulation which stimulates the dermis by bringing in more oxygen and nutrients *Zingiber officinale* (ginger) and *Citrus limon* (lemon).

* The function of the sebaceous glands are effected by *Pelargonium × asperum* (geranium) and *Cymbopogon martinii* (palmarosa). They balance the secretions of these glands as will *Canaga odorata* (ylang ylang). The structure of Jojoba carrier oil also supports the skin's sebum balance.

* All essential oils have some antibacterial activity which will neutralize any pathogenic bacteria and prevent problems from occurring.

* Anti-inflammatory oils, *Chamaemelum nobile* (Roman chamomile) and *Matricaria recutita* (German or blue chamomile) help to reduce many kinds of skin irritation.

* The essential oils reduce stress and tension which often cause skin to look old and taut (you look as old as you feel).

* Carrier oils – Castor and *Rosa rubiginosa* have an effect of improving and supporting the collagen structure of the skin.

The following skin conditions can successfully be treated with aromatherapy:

Acne

Acne caused by excessive secretion of sebum which is controlled by hormonal stimulation from the sex hormones. This is the reason why acne is so often a problem during teenage years and at the premenstrual stage.

Oils that will balance the sebum secretion are for example *Pelargonium* X *asperum* (geranium), *Cymbopogon martinii* (palmarosa), and *Cananga odorata* (ylang ylang).

To avoid the spread of infection use antiseptics of *Juniperus communis* (juniper) or *Cymbopogon martinii* (palmarosa).

Acne rosacea

The cause of Acne rosacea is not known. The condition looks somewhat similar to acne. It is known to cause chronic conjunctivitis of the eyes.

Chamomile flower water will help to reduce the inflammation of the skin as well as ease the conjunctivitis, used on cotton pads over the eyes.

Atopic eczema

This condition is usually found in babies and young children. It often leads to asthma and allergic reactions later in life. In families where there is a tendency to atopic eczema, breast feeding would be the surest way to protect the children, by giving them the necessary immune defences.

The condition can be relieved initially with the use of Evening Primrose oil on the skin, when the baby is very small and also as a food supplement to provide the necessary Gamma Linoleic Acid (GLA).

> "Human breast milk contains GLA and breast-fed babies receive the same amount of GLA found in two to three capsules (1.5 ml) Evening Primrose oil every day"
>
> *Vital Oils*, **Liz Earle**

Further help to the skin can be given by *Chamaemelum nobile* (Roman chamomile) or *Matricaria recutita* (German or blue chamomile) or *Lavandula angustifolia* (lavender) using the dilution suggested according to the age of the child.

Bacterial infections of the skin – Impetigo

This occurs when unwanted bacteria enters areas of damaged skin. For these conditions anti-infectious oils such as *Melaleuca alternifolia, Cymbopogon martinii* or *Thumus vulgaris ct linalol* (thyme) can be successfully used. With any kind of infection it is important that the general wellbeing is improved by helping to boost the immunity, for example by using *Melaleuca alternifolia* (2 drops daily externally) and fighting the infection internally with propolis.

Dermatitis

This is a condition that is caused by a chemical irritation on the skin. The actual reaction can occur immediately upon contact or be delayed up to several days. For this one can use the same soothing oils as above and in future the only answer is to protect oneself from such irritant substances.

Psoriasis

Psoriasis is often hereditary and its causes are not known. The skin cells renew themselves abnormally fast and form a keratinized scaly surface to the affected areas.

Evening Primrose oil internally in high doses (1/2 teaspoon daily) will bring relief to most sufferers, combined with external application of it with 2% *Cymbopogon martinii* (palmarosa) or *Citrus aurantium ssp. bergamia* (bergamot). St. John's Wort maceration also eases the irritation.

Warts

These can be treated with undiluted *Citrus limon* (lemon) or *Melaleuca alternifolia* (tea-tree) oil. One drop directly on the wart 2–3 times daily. It is important to be accurate as both these oils will cause irritation and drying of the skin.

* * * * * *

Other than acne and boils, any new and unusual lumps that grow rapidly or are painful or bleeding must be examined by a medical practitioner before treatment, if any, is applied.

* * * * * *

Daily skin care
Aromatherapy is an excellent daily skin care treatment. Using a facial or body oil based on Jojoba and or Camellia oil will keep skin supple without leaving a greasy feeling or stains on clothes.

The dilution for daily skin care is 0.5–1% and the larger the area used the smaller the percentage.

Scarred skin
Scarred skin from wounds or pregnancy will benefit from daily application of *Rosa rubiginosa* and wheatgerm or hazelnut oils with *Lavandula angustifolia* (lavender) or *Citrus aurantium* flowers (neroli).

OILS FOR THE VARIOUS SKIN TYPES

Dry and sensitive skin:

Matricaria recuitita	German chamomile
Chamaemelum nobile	Roman chamomile
Citrus aurantium flowers	Neroli
Rosa damascena	Rose
Pelargonium × asperum	Geranium
Boswellia carterii	Frankincense
Santalum album	Sandalwood
Cananga odorata	Ylang ylang
Jasminum officinale	Jasmine

Normal skin:

All of those for dry and sensitive skin.
Citrus limon (lemon) is also good but remember photosensitization

Oily skin:

Juniperus communis	Juniper
Cupressus sempervirens	Cypress
Rosmarinus pyramidalis	Rosemary
Cymbopogon martinii	Palmarosa
Citrus aurantium leaves	Petitgrain
Pelargonium × asperum	Geranium
Lavandula angustifolia	Lavender

MENSTRUAL CONDITIONS
The female hormonal system is very delicate and prone to changes and fluctuation for many reasons. It is particularly sensitive to emotional

upsets and upheavals. Over the years a clear pattern has emerged in the treatment of menstrual irregularities and disorders. If no medical problem is apparent, irregular or painful periods can be eased using essential oils that have oestrogen-like effects during the oestrogen phase of the cycle.

Recommended oils are:

> *Salvia sclarea* (clary sage)
> *Melaleuca quinquenervia viridifloral* (niaouli)
> *Artemisia dracunculus* (tarragon)

Others that can be used with caution are

> *Foeniculum vulgare* (fennel)
> *Pimpinella anisum* (aniseed)

THE MENSTRUAL CYCLE

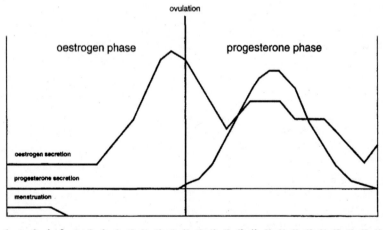

28 day cycle

The same pattern of treatment can be used for PMT, using oestrogen-like oils in the rising, yang phase of the cycle and other oils according to individual needs at the reducing, yin phase of the cycle.

Essential oils for the end of the cycle very often need to have diuretic as well as uplifting properties. Recommended for this *Citrus paradisi* (grapefruit), *Juniperus communis* (juniper), *Citrus aurantium ssp. bergamia* (bergamot). Other oils for the latter part of the cycle to reduce tiredness are *Picea mariana* (black spruce) and *Pinus sylvestris* (pine) and *Chamaemelum nobile* (Roman chamomile) for calming.

Menopausal problems, hot flushes and irritability respond well to the above oestrogen treatment. Two drops of *Cananga odorata* (ylang ylang) applied daily to the lower abdomen and sacrum will ease the hot flushes and simultaneously improve the mucous membrane secretions in the vaginal area, thus relieving the discomfort caused by the dryness.

Hormonal oils are not suitable for treating young girls' painful periods. Their menstrual cycle may not have settled into a regular pattern and oils that influence the hormonal balance may be more harmful than helpful in the long run. A blend of 1 drop lavender, 1 drop *Mentha piperita* (peppermint) and 1 drop *Chamaemelum nobile* (Roman chamomile) will normally bring rapid relief from the discomfort.

All menstrual problems are made worse by stress and tension. Aromatherapy treatments will always reduce the general tension and stress levels so everyone suffering from menstrual disorders of any kind will benefit from aromatherapy.

Evening primrose oil used internally will reduce PMT symptoms in many cases and also help to ease painful breasts.

RHEUMATISM AND ARTHRITIS

Rheumatism is the name given to those undefinable aches and pains, tenderness, inflammation and stiffness in your body. Modern medicine cannot give a reason for the occurrence of these. Natural medicine considers them to be caused by the accumulation of waste matter in the various tissues and the degeneration of cellular metabolism and function.

The real cure for these rheumatic conditions is a cleansing diet of naturally grown food of vegetables, fruit and whole grain cereals. All stimulants such as alcohol, coffee, smoking, tea and chocolate as well as drugs to relieve inflammation and pain, will worsen the situation.

An aromatherapy massage or baths in essential oils that stimulate the elimination of waste and reduce pain help to keep the cleansing process tolerable.

Oils to assist in the cleansing:

> *Rosmarinus pyramidalis* (rosemary)
> *Citrus limon* (lemon)
> *Juniperus communis* (juniper)
> *Thymus vulgaris ct thujanol* (thyme)

To reduce inflammation in the joints:

> *Eucalyptus citriodora* (citrus scented eucalyptus)
> *Betula alleghaniensis* (yellow birch)
> *Helichrysum italicum* (Italian everlasting)

For pain:

> *Laurus nobilis* (bay)
> *Mentha piperita* (peppermint)

Cortisone-like effect on joints:

> *Picea mariana* (black spruce)
> *Pinus sylvestris* (scotch pine)

These oils can all be used as a home treatment massage/rub between aromatherapy treatments.

Arthritis is the follow-up of rheumatism. When waste matter accumulates long enough in large enough quantities, the areas of the body that have the least chance to clear such waste, the joints, begin to suffer, and a chronic, inflammatory, painful condition occurs.

The improvement from this condition is slower and more difficult than from rheumatism, but once again the answer lies in attempting to clear the waste and toxins from the body by dietary measures, and using herbs and essential oils to assist the process. Gentle exercise to keep the joints moving and warming them with compresses and baths ease the discomfort. The congestion of the body in arthritis is difficult to clear. If the aromatherapist does not have sufficient experience in dealing with the dietary aspect of the cleansing, the best approach would be to seek help from a naturopath.

The oils to use in arthritis are the same as for the rheumatic conditions.

9 Hippocratic Temperaments

This section of the book describes the classification of temperament/body types that were first used by Hippocrates (460–377 BC). Right from the very beginning we must remember that these are elements and tendencies that each person holds within themselves and that in an ideal situation they all are held in balance in each of us to create a whole person. Nonetheless there is always one trait which is more dominant than the others and a second one which is clearly definable which then often leaves one trait in the shadow of the temperament.

In aromatherapy we express the importance of taking into account each client's individuality and uniqueness in deciding the essential oils used for each treatment. The following chapters could easily lead into classifying clients into narrow "types" and so it is important to look at this individuality in depth, beyond the text in this book.

I first became acquainted with these temperaments at the Steiner school and day nursery in Turku, Finland. In children the four temperaments are more clearly definable than in adults. It is fascinating to observe the skill with which some of the teachers apply their knowledge of the needs of these characteristics to assist the children in their development and learning.

During development the characteristics go through moulding and changing. In adults the temperaments are more integrated and often environmental and social influences build or inhibit various traits that they can overshadow the natural individuality of the personality.

"Individuality could mean a sum of traits or tendencies collected from the various "types", but these traits are not actually individual but are "typical". In the light of these a human individual then would be concoction of the various influences from each type... Human individuality is deeper than this merging of types. Individuality is the deepest life force, that in growth and development seeks expression, and is unique to everyone... When we respectfully say that someone has personality, we in effect mean, that in him his individuality is allowed to express itself." *(Virkkunen, K., 1981)*

Bilious/Choleric

Personalities whose most dominating features are those found in this type are the people whom we very often meet in situations of leadership. They have a strong desire to be at the head, to take responsibilities, to organise and to give orders. They are strong willed, powerfully energetic and like both physical and psychological effort and activity. They have their "feet on the ground" in BRAVE new ventures or pioneering and have a clearheaded ability to make correct judgements.

When in balance with themselves these people are very charismatic, radiant characters who can hold their authority and audience with ease and assertiveness. They are proud of their achievements and prone to anger when their authority is questioned. On the negative side of the powerfully CHOLERIC type is a possibility of violence and cruelty, fits of temper and uncontrollable rage.

When we look at these personalities at the heads of big business or other demanding jobs and situations we often find that they have stomach ulcers or liver problems. Also their skeletal and muscular systems can become troublesome.

The element of the choleric is fire, which is in constant motion and needs fresh air for healthy life. The types of exercise that suit these powerful strong people are fencing, walking, boxing and extroverted ways of expressing themselves.

The therapist needs to be aware when dealing with the choleric temperament that these people cannot be TOLD anything. They tend to be 'experts' in all areas and need patient persuading to accept that there MAY be some need of change or correction in their lifestyle to benefit their health etc. Patience is also needed as the choleric temperament cannot be hurried or rushed by external influences to reach a decision on anything.

The best approach toward a successful therapy situation, in addition to taking into account the above, is flattery and admiration on the aspects and areas that can HONESTLY be made. Falsity will drive these people away as their respect towards the therapist will then be lost.

The characteristic physical features of the choleric type are large, strong and angular. Their muscles are well formed and hard and can be heavy to work on, skin is matt and feels warm and dry. On the rectangular, square jawed face the expression is dominating, with direct eye contact, and can give an impression of hardness. They have tight lips and abundant, heavy eyebrows. Often the hand seems rectangular, hard and large even in comparison to the usually heavy body. Gestures are wide and vigorous and their walk slow, with long steps.

The fire element dominates the choleric temperament and makes them hot blooded, strong willed persons. They need foods that are cooling and easy on the digestion to assist in bringing balance to the whole being. They need chewing and binding nourishment. Rye and wheat grains, raw root vegetables, water foods such as cucumber and melons of all kinds will cool their ire. They should avoid excessive use of red meats and beans.

The essential oils that are best suited to this temperament when the choleric tendencies have become over-dominating are the cooling, calming oils that contain a lot of aldehydes and esters. These would be, for example, *Eucalyptus citriodora* which also has a property of helping to break out of rigid thought patterns and *Betula alleghaniensis* or *Citrus aurantium petitgrain*, which also assist in the liver functioning.

On the other hand when the choleric person has lost their energy, will and zest, the oils to bring these back are those that contain the dry warming terpenes. Oils such as *Pinus sylvestris*, *Picea mariana* or *Citrus paradisi* could give the necessary lift, depending on the situation.

Sanguine

The first impression given by a person with a dominant sanguine trait is that of someone who likes to be in contact with people, enjoys company and expresses it clearly with welcoming gestures and words. They have an ability to make sharp observations on people and things around them. They are vigorous and optimistic, content with themselves and their achievements. These people have a powerful imagination, are eloquent in their speech and have a deep sense and need of beauty. When the sanguine trait becomes overpowering in a personality the result can be a superficial, complacent person with little or no deep morality.

A predominantly sanguine person has an intense dislike of argument. They are therefore the peacemakers and diplomats, trying to uphold the equilibrium even to the point of their own destruction. They need quiet, calm and affectionate surroundings and loving people around them.

The physiological weaknesses in the heart and arteries reflect this need for love and peace. As the word sanguine itself infers, these people are prone to venous problems such as varicose veins, haemorrhoids, couperose, as well as high blood pressure.

It seems that if a sanguine temperament is undernourished physically or emotionally, or deprived of fresh air they can begin to show signs of the melancholic/nervous temperament.

The element of the sanguine is air and they thrive on fresh air and travelling, and the best form of exercise for them is an outdoor activity that requires both physical and intellectual activity such as orienteering; the sanguine also like to dance.

In the therapy situation the therapist will do well to remember that these people are easily and deeply hurt, though they do not often express it. First and foremost, they need a loving and caring atmosphere and a soft, subtle approach with deep understanding of the fragile inner being that more than anything needs acceptance and love.

The characteristic features of the sanguine physique are well proportioned and give an impression of harmony. Muscles are well formed, tough and wide and when fit, easy and supple to work on. The skin feels moist and warm to touch. The face is oval in shape with reddish complexion, or couperose skin, and a strong full chin. The expression in the eyes is welcoming and mild and lips full and red and their hands are wide and firm.

When expressing themselves in company their gestures are numerous, quick and wide and their walk quick with long steps.

The foods that will help to 'gather' the sanguine person together are nuts and almonds. Vegetarian diet helps concentration by grounding the emotions, and occasional eggs or meat will help to keep the sanguine person 'on the earth'. Herbs can also be used to help the metabolism.

Essential oils that help the sanguine keep their feet on the ground contain esters or sesquiterpenes. *Chamaemelum nobile* or *Matricaria recutita* are good examples of these, as is *Helichrysum italicum*. When we look at the weak areas of this temperament, oils that help to lower blood pressure or support the circulatory system are also very useful. These are, for example, *Citrus limon*, *Lavandula angustifolia* (high esters), *Cananga odorata* and *Cupressus sempervirens*.

At the other end of the scale, when the sanguine have been deprived of the right kind of nourishment at any level and have turned to melancholia, they need warming by essential oils that contain a good proportion of monoterpenic alcohols or even phenols. The oils suitable for this are *Origanum majorana*, *Citrus aurantium neroli*, *Thymus vulgaris ct. linalol* or *Thujanol* and also possibly *Santalum album* for the emotional warming of the sacral area.

Lymphatic/Phlegmatic

The calm, sedentary lymphatic type likes peace and tranquillity and a regular lifestyle. They are at their best in repetitive tasks and in a fairly slow tempo.

They take a long time to 'get started' but when they do, they are patient and reliable in whatever they do. They have an inborn sense of reality and are able to look at an ideal with clarity. On the negative side of this temperament is a great resistance to change, laziness and boredom. They can become dreamers and be inconsistent in their dealings.

The physical appearance of the lymphatic reflects their love of food and they tend to be overweight. Their musculature is soft and not clearly defined and skin is white and feels cold and moist to touch.

The element of the lymphatic temperament is water, which has an effect of slowing down activity. Their weak areas are related to this liquidity and they tend to suffer from fluid retention and problems in the endocrine system. They also often have problems in the digestive area.

The people with the lymphatic temperament predominating need to have stimulating physical and mental activity and environment.

In a therapeutic situation one must remember that these people cannot be hurried, and out of balance have a resistance to change in many levels. They need to be treated gently but with authority, respecting their need to take time to ponder over new matters before even attempting any change.

Their round or almost pearshaped faces often appear expressionless with lips that are full and pale. Verbal expression is slow and gestures rare and they walk with slow and short steps.

Food is the subject that brings a phlegmatic person alive and correct types of food can be used to stimulate and awaken them. Acid foods, sauerkraut or apple cider vinegar pickles and warming herbs and spices are very appropriate. The dreamy phlegmatic should avoid potatoes or milk in excess.

The essential oils to stimulate and activate phlegmatic people are those that contain mainly monoterpenes and have diuretic or drying and warming effect, such as *Juniperus communis*, *Citrus paradisi*, *Zingiber officinale*, *Pinus sylvestris* and *Picea mariana*.

Pelargonium × asperum, *Cupressus sempervirens* and *Pogostemon cablin* are oils that will assist the lymphatic function and are therefore useful for this temperament, and *Mentha piperita* and *Citrus limon* will stimulate the digestive system.

Melancholic/Nervous

The fragile looking, timid melancholics are often very artistic. They prefer mental activity and like to spend time in solitary work researching or on arts. They have an innovative mind and clarity in drawing conclusions. In their dealings with people they are honest and scrupulous. Their intuitive and curious nature is easily impressed by outside influences which then can cause anxiety and agitation. On the negative side of this temperament is difficulty in adapting to new situations, inconsistency in action and irregularity, making time-keeping for example difficult to stick to.

The nervous system is the weakest link in the physique of this temperament. They also have a fragile immune system and are prone to chronic infections which, if allowed to continue too long, can go deep into the skeleton and create problems there.

The element of the melancholic is earth. They are thinkers, easily depressed and tend to curl up in their shell. They need optimistic, calm surroundings and stimulating mental activity. Fresh air and physical exercise and a good rhythm to their daily activities are vital to the wellbeing of melancholic type.

In the therapeutic situation the therapist needs to know her subject in depth and be prepared to explain, discuss and reason through all of the treatment, to make a therapeutic situation that is most beneficial to the melancholic client.

The physiological features of the melancholic temperament give an impression of being fragile, wiry or angular and frail, their muscles are knotted, narrow and unyielding and skin is yellowish, dry and cold. The face is triangular in shape with deepset, restless eyes, thin lips and narrow chin.

The gestures of the melancholic temperament are quick and ceaseless and the walk quick with short steps. The verbal expression is rapid and intermittent.

The melancholic people need taste experiences that will give them pleasure, warmth and light. Sun-ripened sweet fruits such as raisins and honey, grains of barley and oats, and red beetroots and carrots are suitable. To bring the heat and fire of the choleric temperament into the coolness of the melancholic, spices like paprika, pepper, curry or mustard are the answer.

Essential oils for these people when the melancholy is overtaking need to be the warming, anti-infectious monoterpenic alcohols or phenols as at the down times their immune defences are at their very lowest. In this category are first included *Thymus vulgaris ct. linalol* or *thujano*, *Melaleuca alternifolia* for its immunostimulant properties and *Cymbopogon martinii* as it supports the nervous system in addition to its anti-infectious activity. The melancholic physique feels the cold easily and warming oils such as *Origanum majorana* or *Zingiber officianale* will feel comforting.

If the lifestyle of the melancholic person does not allow regularity and rhythm it can result in over anxiety, agitation and insecurity with fears and lack of self-confidence. *Jasminum officinale* and *Santalum album* can bring light and strength and help to overcome these overwhelming feelings.

BALANCING THE HIPPOCRATIC TEMPERAMENTS USING THE COMPOSITION OF THE ESSENTIAL OILS

Phlegmatic/ Lymphatic	Melancholic/ Nervous
Needs monoterpenes *to warm and stimulate lymphatic* *function and remove fluids*	*Needs alcohols, phenols* *to boost immune system* *to warm and strengthen*
ESTERS	
ALDEHYDES	
KETONES	
	SESQUI- TERPENES
ALCOHOLS	
PHENOLS	MONOTERPENES
Sanguine	Choleric/ Bilious
Needs esters, sesquiterpenes *to lower blood pressure* *and calm and reduce inflammation*	*Needs aldehydes, ketones, esters* *to calm and cool* *to assist liver function*

Madam Maury described these balancing effects of essential oils as follows:

"To reduce the excesses and strengthen the areas of weakness"

For example, if a person of the nervous temperament is so out of balance and deep in melancholy that he suffers from a chronic infection, he needs the warming, stimulating, anti-infectious and immunity boosting properties of the alcohols and phenols. On the other hand, if the world has disturbed the energy of the melancholic so much that his creativity and inner life is fading, he needs the calming effect of the esters and sesquiterpenes.

QUICK REFERENCE CHART OF THE GENERAL APPEARANCE FOR THE HIPPOCRATIC TEMPERAMENTS

Hippocratic Temperament	Bilious/Choleric	Nervous – Melancholic	Sanguine	Lymphatic – Phlegmatic
CHARACTERISTIC FEATURES	Massive/angular	Angular/frail	Roundshaped firm	Roundshaped flabby
WALK	Long steps/slow	Short steps/ quick	Long steps/ quick	Short steps/ slow
GESTURES	Wide/vigorous	Quick/ceaseless	Wide/numerous/ quick	Rare/slow
MUSCLES	Hard/long/well shaped	Frail/knotted	Wide/tough/ well shaped	No real outline
SPEECH	Assertive	Quick/jerky	Quick/easy	Slow
FACE	Rectangular	Triangle	Oval	Pear-shaped
COMPLEXION	Matt	Yellowish	Reddish	White
SKIN	Dry/warm	Dry/cold	Warm/wet	Cold/wet
EYEBROWS	Abundant	Sparse	Abundant	Sparse
LOOK	Straight/ dominating/hard	Unfixed/deep set	Laughing/ welcoming/mild	Expressionless
NOSE	Square	Thin/pointed	Straight/ upturned	Square
LIPS	Straight	Thin	Full/red	Full/white
CHIN	Wide	Thin/narrow	Full/strong	Double
HAND	Rectangular/hard	Triangular/thin	Hexagonal/firm/ wide	White/large/ flabby/wet

10 *The Therapist*

ESSENTIAL OILS

Undoubtedly the therapist will be influenced and affected by the essential oils she uses for the treatments. The oils will be absorbed through her hands and respiration and they will also have an effect through the sense of smell.

Using good quality, pure essential oils there should be no problems, but it is good to remember and respect the basic rules and precautions.

It is possible to be allergic to some of the essential oils, especially the citrus oils, but allergic reactions even to these can be caused not so much by the oil itself, but the residues of the preservative or the pesticide sprays that can be left in the cold-pressed essence.

The therapist must also listen to herself when using and choosing the essential oils for her clients. They should not feel or smell unpleasant for the therapist either. If they do they should not be used and other oils chosen. A therapist giving a treatment whilst feeling headachey or nauseous will not benefit the client.

Changing the oils from one client to the next in the course of the day avoids the cumulative effect of the individual oils on the therapist.

It is possible to become used and attached to using a set of oils. Every so often it is worth having a look at the essential oil repertoire and finding alternatives to those that are used most regularly to enable the senses and body systems to have a break from them for a while.

The dosages used must be respected, remembering that the essential oils have an effect on the physical, and the energetic aspects of both the client and the therapist.

In aromatherapy 'more is not necessarily better'.

THE CARRIER OILS

The quality of the carrier oils is as important as the quality of the essential oils. They need to be cold pressed, and processed, deodorized etc. as little as possible.

The carrier oils do not have an effect on the therapist in the same way as the essential oils. Good quality carrier oils do, however, improve the condition of the skin on the therapist's hands and sweet almond oil in particular will strengthen the nails. Sometimes one finds that the skin on the face may also feel oilier at the end of many treatments.

It is worth noting that those allergic to some tree pollens can also have allergic reactions to nut oils.

WORKING POSTURE

Even light massage performed all day is physically demanding and using one's body in a way that preserves energies is a matter of posture and technique. For the correct working posture the table height must be 'tailor made' for the therapist and the space around needs to be big enough for free movement and working from all sides of the table.

The most beneficial massage techniques for the client and the best for the therapist's own balance – physical and mental – are ones that work equally and in the same way from both sides of the body and table. Initially it means that the therapist has to learn to use the less active hand in the same way as the other. This, though awkward at first, is doubly beneficial. It helps both sides of the therapist's brain to a more equal functioning, and ensures that the muscles are used in the same way on both sides of the body. In this way the therapist is also 'treated' towards balance whilst treating, and a lot of tiredness is avoided.

LOOKING AFTER ONESELF

The therapist needs to look after herself both physically and emotionally to give her best to each and every client. None of us are superhuman or angels, however much we wish we were.

To be able to give from one's heart, one needs to learn to receive. The therapist needs treatments. In working full-time, a weekly treatment is recommended, but not necessarily aromatherapy. Any treatment that allows a relaxation of the body and rest for the mind is fine, providing there is good rapport and understanding between the client and the therapist.

Taking a clear break and learning to let go between clients by giving oneself enough time to have a drink and 'breathe' for a few moments is vital. If this is not learned one can 'carry' all the day's clients with oneself to the evening. There are many methods for this. A simple visualization of separating oneself and the client into individual orbs of light is very effective and takes only a little while.

The therapist carrying the client's problems will not help them. It leads to the therapist being exhausted and unable to find peace. The answers to each client's problems are always within themselves and cannot be solved from outside. The wise therapist learns to listen wisely without absorbing the client's heartaches and sorrows. Often it is enough for the client to talk out the problems, and while doing so the answers appear from within.

The therapist can feel all alone in her own profession and a therapy group locally would be beneficial to all those taking part in it. These give a chance of giving and receiving support from the other local practitioners as therapists and as individuals.

GROWING AS A THERAPIST

Growing as a therapist can be seen in the light of very practical aspects of learning more of one's profession by keeping up with studies and findings, and growing spiritually to fulfil the clients' needs better. It also could mean to follow one's personal path in this profession which in its essence is working for the wellbeing of man and the earth.

The practical growing occurs naturally in the working situation where each client in their uniqueness presents a new challenge and a new learning situation to work with.

Courses of many descriptions and subjects touching and supporting aromatherapy can be found in the many aromatherapy organizations. Finding the right route for oneself can at first be a hit and miss affair. Qualifying as an aromatherapist, or any other therapist, usually gives such a thirst for learning more that many new therapists go on a continuous race of courses on various subjects. This leads into not having time to deepen and strengthen that which is already learned, and weakening and clouding the knowledge. To keep on the fairly 'straight and narrow' seems to be the answer in the end for many therapists.

Undoubtedly it is good to know and understand enough of the various complementary therapies. This enables the therapist to guide those clients that she is not able to treat to some other more suitable therapist.

Growing and strengthening spiritually as a therapist is a continuous process throughout the working life. The most difficult and most rewarding task is to learn to respect and love each client as they are, each time they come to be treated; respecting their rights and gently guiding them into taking responsibility for their own health and wellbeing without imposing our own will upon their progress. The client may well be a 'good girl' and do all that is asked of her, but feel that it is not suitable for her, and therefore the benefit gained from the treatment will be short lived when the new routine stops, as there is no therapist 'checking on it'.

Growing as a therapist is also a continuous inner change, particularly if treatments are also received as well as given. Physical and spiritual practices such as yoga, tai-chi, walking etc. are times of self cleansing and concentration during which a deeper understanding of oneself begins. They also help in improving concentration on the task at hand, which is necessary to be able to be 'with the client' throughout the treatment without letting the mind wander onto other matters.

Learning to breathe freely whilst treating is partly a matter of working posture and partly of awareness during the treatment. This awareness can be described as being in tune with the free flow of one's own energies; being aware that one is not a closed circuit, but in a stream of continuous exchange of many forms of energy within and without ones own body. In this way the work does not tire the therapist and is very invigorating and strengthening for the client. This does not mean any so called 'willed energy transfer' from the therapist to the client, but understanding that there is a continuous movement of energies in the treatment situation. Working with will from one's own limited energy resources surely tires the therapist in the long term.

Spiritual growth does not happen in the head but it develops from a combination of both physical and mental work; strengthening and cleansing one's physical body is essential groundwork for being able to 'understand in the body' what is gained intellectually from spiritual teachers or from books.

This 'understanding in the body' could be called the intuitive knowledge or sensing of other peoples needs. It is not however imagination.

"So easily in this age of newly found spirituality we let our imagination run riot."

Here is a very sobering thought from a Canadian polarity therapy teacher, Howard Kiewe, who has his feet firmly placed on the ground, but his integrity touches the heavens. He teaches his students not to assume anything from external happenings or signs and waits for the client himself to express his feelings and emotions. He says:

"Tears in your clients eyes are not necessarily a sign of deep emotional release or experience – they may well be caused by the fact that you have just been working on some area that is physically very painful."

Here on this earth, in this physical world, everything must come to our understanding, awareness and cognition through the physical body. It is our tool for spiritual growth – the pains, the joys and sorrows of our soul we feel in our physical being. As a holistic therapist we treat our clients' physical body – helping the body to heal the wounds that life has caused. At the same time we must remember that these same holistic facts of life apply to us as growing therapists.

In conclusion an old Finnish saying:

"A healthy soul, in a healthy body, will allow the free expression of the spirit, of the light of which we all are a spark."

11 *Terminology*

GENERAL TERMINOLOGY

ABSOLUTE
A highly concentrated viscous, semi-solid or solid perfume material, usually obtained by alcohol extraction from the concrete.

ALLERGY
Hypersensitivity caused by a foreign substance, small doses of which produce a violent bodily reaction.

AMENORRHOEA
Absence of menstruation.

ANAEMIA
Deficiency in either quality of quantity of red corpuscles in the blood.

ANATOMY
Refers to the location of the parts in relation to the rest of the body.

ANOREXIA
Condition of being without, or having lost the appetite for food.

APOPLEXY
Sudden loss of consciousness, a stroke or sudden severe haemorrhage.

ARTHRITIS
Inflammation of a joint or joints.

ASTHENIA
Weakness, lack of tone.

BILIOUS
A condition caused by an excessive secretion of bile.

CARDIAC
Pertaining to the heart.

CATARRH
Inflammation of mucous membranes, usually associated with an increase in secretion of mucus.

CELL
Term first used by Robert Hook (1665). It is the 'basic building block'. Cells have different sizes, shapes, contents and functions. Cells with similar physical characteristics normally carry out a similar function.

CELLULITE
Accumulation of toxic matter in the tissue fluids.

CEREBRAL
Pertaining to the largest part of the brain, the cerebrum.

CHEMOTYPE
Variation of main chemical components within a species due to growing conditions.

CHOLESTEROL
A steroid alcohol found in nervous tissue, red blood cells, animal fat and bile.

CIRRHOSIS
Degenerative change in an organ (especially the liver) caused by various poisons, bacteria or other agents, resulting in fibrous tissue overgrowth.

COLIC
Pain due to contraction of the involuntary muscle of the abdominal organs.

COLITIS
Inflammation of the colon.

COMPRESS
A lint or substance applied hot or cold to an area of the body, for relief of swelling or pain, or to produce localized pressure.

CONCRETE
A concentrated, waxy, solid or semi-solid perfume material prepared from previously live plant matter, usually using a hydrocarbon solvent.

CONSTIPATION
Congestion of the bowels; incomplete or infrequent action of the bowels.

CUTANEOUS
Pertaining to the skin.

CYSTITIS
Bladder inflammation, usually characterized by pain on urinating.

DEBILITY
Weakness, lack of tone.

DECOCTION
A herbal preparation made by boiling the plant material for 10–20 minutes, starting with cold water.

DERMAL
Pertaining to the skin.

DERMATITIS
Inflammation of the skin; many causes.

DIARRHOEA
Frequent passage of unformed liquid bowels.

DYSMENORRHOEA
Painful and difficult menstruation.

DYSPEPSIA
Difficulty with digestion associated with pain, flatulence, heartburn and nausea.

ENTERITIS
Inflammation of the mucous membrane of the intestine.

ENZYME
Complex proteins that are produced by living cells, and catalyze specific biochemical reactions.

EXTERNAL ENVIRONMENT
Refers to that which is outside the body.

GASTRITIS
Inflammation of stomach lining.

GENITO-URINARY
Referring to both the genital and the reproductive systems.

GINGIVITIS
Inflammation of the gums, manifested by swelling and bleeding.

HALITOSIS
Offensive breath.

HAEMORRHOIDS
Piles, dilated rectal veins.

HEARTWOOD
The central portion of a tree trunk.

HEPATIC
Relating to the liver (tones and aids its function).

HERBAL EXTRACT
A more concentrated preparation, made by the maceration process. Usually used as drops diluted in water or other liquids.

HERBAL OIL
An oil prepared by steeping the plant material in a bland oil.

HERPES
Inflammation of the skin or mucous membrane with clusters of deep-seated vesicles.

HORMONE
A substance secreted by specialized cells, which controls specific tissues or processes within the body.

HYPERTENSION
Raised blood pressure.

HYPOTENSION
Low blood pressure, or a fall in blood pressure below the normal range.

INFUSION
A herbal preparation made by pouring boiling water on the fresh or dried herb (as for teas).

INSOMNIA
Inability to sleep.

INTERNAL ENVIRONMENT
Refers to that which is **inside** the body.

LEUCOCYTE
White blood cells responsible for fighting disease.

LEUCORRHEA
White discharge from the vagina.

LYMPHATIC
Pertaining to the lymph system.

MACERATION
A herbal preparation made by steeping the plant material at room temperature for hours or days. The liquid may be water, alcohol, wine or oil.

MENOPAUSE
The normal cessation of menstruation, a life change for women.

MENORRHAGIA
Excessive menstruation.

MICROBE
A minute living organism, especially pathogenic bacteria, viruses, etc.

NEPHRITIS
Inflammation of the kidneys.

NEURALGIA
A stabbing pain along a nerve pathway.

OEDEMA
A painless swelling caused by fluid retention beneath the skin's surface.

OESTROGEN
A hormone produced by the ovary, necessary for the development of the female secondary sexual characteristics.

OLFACTION
The sense of smell.

ORGAN
Composed of a number of different tissues which all help perform its specific task.

OTITIS
Inflammation of the ear.

PALPITATION
Undue awareness of the heartbeat.

PATHOLOGICAL
Unnatural or destructive process on living tissue.

PEPTIC
Applied to gastric secretions and areas affected by them.

PHARMACOLOGY
Medical science of drugs which deals with their actions, properties and characteristics.

PHARMACOPOEIA
An official publication of drugs in common use, in a given country.

PHYSIOLOGICAL
Describes the natural biological processes of a living organism.

PHYTOHORMONES
Plant substances that mimic the action of human hormones.

PHYTOTHERAPY
The treatment of disease by plants; herbal medicine.

PROSTATITIS
Any inflammatory condition of the prostate gland.

PRURITIS
Itching

PSORIASIS
A skin disease characterized by red patches and silver scaling.

PULMONARY
Pertaining to the lungs.

PYORRHOEA
Bleeding or a discharge of pus.

RECITIFICATION
The process of redistillation applied to essential oils to rid them of certain constituents.

RENAL
Pertaining to the kidney.

RHINITIS
Inflammation of the mucous membrane of the nose.

SCIATICA
Pain down the back of the legs, in the area supplied by the sciatic nerve, due to various causes including pressure on the nerve roots.

SCLEROSIS
Hardening of tissue due to inflammation.

SEBORRHOEA
Increased secretion of sebum, usually associated with excessive oily secretion from the sweat glands.

SYSTEM
Composed of a number of different organs and tissues. Each system carries out a precise, vital function to enable the body to survive. Each system should work in harmony with the others to bring about a balanced internal environment. Each system satisfies a specific need of the body.

TACHYCARDIA
Abnormally increased heartbeat and pulse rate.

THROMBOSIS
Formation of a thrombus or blood clot.

THRUSH
An infection of the mouth or vaginal region caused by a fungus (Candida).

TINCTURE
A clear, coloured liquid prepared by macerating the plant material in alcohol, pressing and finally filtering.

TISSUES
A large number of cells closely associated and performing the same specialized function.

URTICARIA
Hives, nettle rash, acute or chronic affection of the skin characterized by the formation of weals, attended by itching, stinging or burning.

UTERINE
Pertaining to the uterus.

VOLATILE
Unstable, evaporates easily, as in 'volatile oil'.

GLOSSARY OF TERMS USED TO DESCRIBE THE PROPERTIES OF ESSENTIAL OILS

ANAESTHETIC	Loss of feeling or sensation; substance which causes such loss.
ANALGESIC	Remedy or agent which deadens pain.
ANAPHRODISIAC	Decreasing sexual desire.
ANTHELMINTIC	Expelling intestinal worms.
ANTIBIOTIC	Prevents the growth of, or destroys, bacteria.
ANTICARIOUS	Preventing decay of teeth.
ANTICATARRHAL	An agent which helps remove excess catarrh from the body.
ANTICONVULSIVE	Preventing convulsions.
ANTIDEPRESSANT	Helps alleviate depression.
ANTIHISTAMINE	Treats allergic conditions; counteracts effects of histamine.
ANTIHYPERTENSIVE	Preventing the occurrence of high blood pressure.

ANTI-INFLAMMATORY	Reduces inflammation.
ANTILITHIC	Prevents the formation of a calculus or stone.
ANTIMICROBIAL	An agent which resists or destroys pathogenic micro-organisms.
ANTINEURALGIC	Relieves and reduces nerve pain.
ANTIPHLOGISTIC	Checks or counteracts inflammation.
ANTIPRURITIC	Relieves sensation of itching or prevents its occurrence.
ANTIRHEUMATIC	Helps prevent or remove rheumatism.
ANTISCLEROTIC	Helps prevent the hardening of tissue.
ANTISEBORRHOEIC	Helps control the production of sebum, the oily secretion from sweat glands.
ANTISEPTIC	Destroys and prevents the spreading of microbes.
ANTISPASMODIC	Prevents and eases spasms or convulsions.
ANTISUDORIFIC	Antiperspirant, reduces perspiration.
ANTITOXIC	Counteracting poisons.
ANTIVIRAL	Substance which inhibits the growth of a virus.
APHRODISIAC	Increases or stimulates sexual desire.
ASTRINGENT	Causing constriction of tissues locally.
BACTERICIDE	An agent that destroys bacteria.
BACTERIOSTATIC	Inhibits growth of bacteria.
BECHIC	An agent that promotes or induces coughing.
CALMATIVE	A sedative.
CARDIOTONIC	Having a stimulating effect on the heart.
CARMINATIVE	Settles the digestive system, eases colic and flatulence.

CEPHALIC	Remedy for disorders of the head; referring or directed towards the head.
CHOLAGOGIC	Stimulating the flow of bile into the duodenum by contraction of the gall bladder.
CHOLERETIC	Increasing the secretion of bile by the liver.
CICATRICANT	Promoting healing by the formation of scar tissue.
CORDIAL	A tonic for the heart.
CYTOPHYLACTIC	An agent that assists any cellular defensive system that serves to protect against an attack by injurious agents, particularly infective organisms.
CYTOTOXIC	Toxic to all cells.
DECONGESTANT	Helps to diminish catarrhal blockage e.g. in the nose.
DEODORANT	An agent which corrects, masks or removes unpleasant odours.
DEPURATIVE	Cleansing, particularly in relating to purifying the blood.
DIAPHORETIC	Promoting sweating/sudorific.
DIGESTIVE	Substance which promotes or aids the digestion of food.
DISINFECTANT	Prevents and combats the spread of germs.
DIURETIC	Aids production of urine, promotes urination, increases flow.
EMETIC	Induces vomiting.
EMMENAGOGUE	Induces or assists menstruation.
EMOLLIENT	Softens and soothes the skin.
EXPECTORANT	Helps removal of phlegm and catarrh from the respiratory system.

FEBRIFUGE	Helps reduce fever/antipyretic.
FUNGICIDE	Prevents and combats fungal infection.
GALACTOGOGUE	Promotes the flow of breast-milk.
GERMICIDAL	Destroys germs or micro-organisms such as bacteria, etc.
HAEMOSTATIC	Stops bleeding.
HALLUCINOGENIC	Causes visions or delusions.
HYPERTENSIVE	Raises blood pressure.
HYPNOTIC	Induces sleep.
HYPOTENSIVE	Lowers blood pressure.
IMMUNOSTIMULANT	Strengthens the body's resistance to infection.
INSECTICIDE	Repels insects.
LAXATIVE	Promotes evacuation of the bowels.
LIPOLYTIC	Breaking down fats.
LITHOLYTIC	Dissolving of stones e.g. bladder.
MUCOLYTIC	Dissolving or breaking down mucus.
NERVINE	A nerve tonic.
PARTURIENT	Aids childbirth.
PARASITICIDE	Prevents and destroys parasites such as fleas, lice, etc.
PATHOGENIC	Causing or producing disease.
PURGATIVE	A substance stimulating an evacuation of the bowels.
RELAXANT	Soothing, causing relaxation, relieving strain or tension.
RUBEFACIENT	A substance which causes redness of the skin, possibly irritation.

SEDATIVE	An agent which reduces functional activity; calming.
SOPORIFIC	A substance which induces sleep.
SPASMOLYTIC	See antispasmodic.
SPLENETIC	Strengthening or tonifying the spleen.
STIMULANT	An agent which quickens the physiological functions of the body.
STOMACHIC	Digestive aid and tonic; improving appetite.
SUDORIFIC	Promoting perspiration.
TONIC	Strengthens and enlivens the whole or specific parts of the body.
UTERINE	Giving tone to the uterus.
VASOCONSTRICTOR	Causing constriction of blood vessels either locally or generally.
VASODILATOR	Dilates the blood vessels.
VERMIFUGE	Eliminating intestinal worms.
VULNERARY	An agent which helps heal wounds and sores by external application.

12 *Hazardous Essential Oils*

The following essential oils present risks, either of toxicity, skin irritation, and/or skin sensitization. They are therefore, not considered safe in general use.

List by the International Federation of Aromatherapists.

COMMON NAME	LATIN NAME
Almond (bitter)	*Prunus amygdalus var. amara*
Boldo lead	*Peumus boldus*
Calamus	*Acorus calamus*
Camphor (brown)	*Cinnamomum camphora*
Camphor (yellow)	
Cassia	*Cinnamomum aromaticum*
Cinnamon bark	*Cinnamomum verum zeylanicum*
Clove bud	*Eugenia caryophyll*
Clove leaf	*Eugenia caryophyll*
Clove stem	*Eugenia caryophyll*
Costus	*Saussurea lappa*
Elecampane	*Inula helenium*
Fennel (bitter)	*Foeniculum vulgare var vulgare*
Horseradish	*Cochlearia armorica*
Jaborandi leaf	*Pilocarpus jaborandi*
Mugwort (armoise)	*Artemisia vulgaris*
Mustard (black)	*Brassica nigra*
Oregano	*Origanum vulgare*
Origanum (Spanish)	*Thymus capitatus*
Pennyroyal (European)	*Mentha pulegium*
Pennyroyal (N. American)	*Hedeoma pulegioides*
Pine (Dwarf)	*Pinus pumilio*
Rue	*Ruta graveolens*
Sassafras	*Sassafras albidum*
Sassafras (Brazilian)	*Ocotea cymbarum*
Savin	*Juniperus sabina*
Savory (summer)	*Satureja hortensis*

Savory (winter)	*Satureja montana*
Southernwood	*Artemisia abrotanum*
Tansy	*Tanacetum vulgare*
Thuja (cedar leaf)	*Thuja occidentalis*
Thuja plicata	*Thuja plicata*
Wintergreen	*Gaultheria procumbens*
Wormseed	*Chenopodium ambrosiodes anthelminticum*
Wormwood	*Artemisia absinthium*

Bibliography

Arponen, R., Valtonen, E., **Hieronta Opas ja Käsikirja**, Werner Söderströn Ltd., Porvoo, Finland, 1982

Ball, J., **Understanding Disease**, The C.W. Daniel Co. Ltd., Saffron Walden, United Kingdom, 1993

Balz, R., **Les Huiles Essentielles et Comment les Utiliser**, L'Imprimerie du Crestois, Crest, France, 1986

Davis, P., **Aromatherapy An A–Z**, The C.W. Daniel Co. Ltd., Saffron Walden, United Kingdom, 1988

Davis, P., **Subtle Aromatherapy**, The C.W. Daniel Co. Ltd., Saffron Walden, United Kingdom, 1992

Earle, L., **Vital Oils**, Ebury Press, London, United Kingdom, 1991

Franchome, P., Penoel, D., **L'Aromaterapie Exactement**, Roger Jollois Editeur, Limoges, France, 1990

Gumbel, D., **Gesunde Haut mit Heilkräuter-Essenzen**, Karl F. Haug Verlag GmbH & Co., Heidelberg, Germany, 1984

Hervonen, A., **Tuki ja Liikuntaelimistön Anatomia**, Lääketiteteellinen Oppimateriaalikustantamo, Ltd., Tampere, Finland, 1992

Hiltunen, R., Holm Y., **Luonnonlääkkeet**, University of Helsinki, Helsinki, Finland, 1994

Holm, Y., **Headspace Gas Chromatography in the Analysis of Volatile Oils**, Yvonne Holm, Helsinki, Finland, 1990

Lassak & McCarthy, **Australian Medicinal Plants**, Mandarin, Australia, 1990

Lawles, J., **The Encyclopaedia of Essential Oils**, Element Books Ltd., Dorset, United Kingdom, 1992

Lindberg, M., **Lapin ja Pohjois-Suomen Rhodos ja Luontaistuotekasveista**, Kuopio University Publications, Kuopio, Finland, 1993.

Mansfield, P., **The Good Health Handbook**, Grafton Books, London, United Kingdom, 1988

Maury, M., **Marguerite Maury's Guide to Aromatherapy; The Secret of Life and Youth**, The C.W. Daniel Co. Ltd., Saffron Walden, United Kingdom, 1989

Nienstedt et al., **Ihmisen Fysiologia ja Anatomia**, Wener Söderström Ltd., Porvoo, Finland, 1989

Peräsalo, J., **Sisätautioppi**, Wener Söderström Ltd., Porvoo, Finland, 1990

Rautavaara, T., **Miten Luonto Parantaa**, Werner Söderström Ltd., Porvoo, Finland, 1980

Van Dam, J., **Parantavat Voimat Ihmisessä ja Yhteisössä**, Finnish Antroposofic Union, Helsinki, Finland, 1991

Virkkunen, K., **Temperamentit**, Antroposofic Work Centre, Tampere, Finland, 1981

Williams, D., **Lecture Notes on Essential Oils**, Eve Taylor (London) Ltd., London, United Kingdom, 1989

ARTICLES AND LECTURE NOTES

Hiltunen, R., Holm, Y. Lecture Notes, Helsinki, 1995

Jeal, W., Lecture notes on Anatomy and Physiology, 1992–1994

Rautajoki, A., Terapeuttinen Kosketus-Käsitteen analyysi ja Uudelleen-määrittely, 1993

Index

Essential oils are indexed under both their English and Latin names except where these would appear consecutively when only the Latin name is listed (e.g. Angelica).

A
abbreviations, 14
abscess, 74, 84 *and see* cellulitis
absolute, definition, 150
absorption rates, 110
aches *see* headaches, muscles, pain
Achillea liquistica (Yarrow), 1, 77
acid, 16
acne
    hydrolats for, 84, 85
    oils for, 25, 34, 47, 48, 59, 60, 63, 71, 131
    and see acne rosacea, skin
acne rosacea, 47, 131 *and see* acne, skin
activity, and skin temperature, 112
adenoids, 36, 113, 123 *and see* nose
adrenal insufficiency, 71
ageing, combating, 83
agitation, 25 *and see* anxiety
air conditioning, and skin, 113
alcohol, 15, 113
aldehyde, 16
allergies, 47, 64, 145, 146, 150
Almond Oil (Sweet), 82
alveoli, 114
amenorrhoea, 29, 31, 37, 150
    and see menstrual problems

anaemia, 111, 150 *and see* blood
anatomy, definition, 150
anethole, 17
Angelica archangelica (Angelica), 22, 79
angelisine, 17
anger, 79
Aniba rosaeodora (Rosewood), 13, 68–9, 79, 124, 126
anorexia, 22, 30, 150 *and see* appetite loss
anosmia, 116
anxiety, 1, 22, 23, 26, 30, 47, 53, 79, 80, 121 *and see* agitation, nerves
aphrodisiacs, 70
apoplexy, definition, 150
appetite loss, 24, 42 *and see* anorexia
appointment records, 101–2
Apricot Kernel oil, 82
Arnot-Schultz rule, 92
aromatherapy
    cosmetic, 5
    effects of, 6, 7–8
    history, 1–4
    points to note, 18–20
    therapeutic, 5–6
    triangle of, 7

Lemon (*Citrus limon*), 49–50, 115,
121, 122, 128, 129, 130, 132,
136, 140, 141
leucocyte, definition, 154
leucorrhea, definition, 154
ligaments, sprained, 71
Ling, P.E., 86
Linneaus, Carolus (Carl von
Linné), 3
liver, 49, 59
stimulant, 41, 56
and see hepatitis, jaundice
lumbago, 70
lungs, 92, 112, 114 *and see*
pleurisy, respiratory system
lymph system, 41, 93, 130, 154
lymphatic temperament, 140–1

M
Macadamia Nut oil, 83
maceration, 154
Mandarin (*Citrus reticulata*), 51–2,
80, 129
Marjoram (*Origanum majorana*),
1, 52–3, 120, 121, 122, 123,
140, 142
massage, 86–7
physiological effects, 91–4
strokes, 87–90
as treatment, 100–1
and see therapeutic touch
Matricaria recutita (German/Blue
Chamomile), 29, 126, 130, 131,
140
Maury, Marguerite, 4
medication, 18, 113
medicine, aromatic, 5
Melaleuca alternifolia (Tea-Tree),

1, 74–5, 122, 123, 126, 127,
130, 132, 142
Melaleuca quinquenervia (Niaouli),
58–9, 128
melancholic temperament, 141–3
Melissa officinalis (Melissa), 2, 80,
85, 121
menopause, 32, 37, 78, 135, 154
menorrhagia, 154 *and see*
menstrual problems
menstrual problems, 41, 59, 121,
133–5 *and see* amenorrhoea,
dysmenorrhoea, menorrhagia,
periods, PMT
Mentha piperita (Peppermint),
61–2, 120, 122, 123, 126, 129,
135, 136, 141
metabolism, and massage, 93
methyl-ether, 17
microbe, definition, 154
migraine, 62 *and see* headaches
mind, 105
moisture, and skin, 113
molecule groups, 14–18
moles, pigmentation reduction, 35
monoterpene, 15
mood swings, 26, 47, 79
mouth
infections, 25, 127
ulcers, 55, 127
and see gum infections, teeth
multiple sclerosis, 60 *and see* sclerosis
muscles
aching, 30, 42, 53, 73
congested, 47
fatigued, 66
inflamed, 30
and massage, 93–4